THERAPEUTIC APHERESIS: A PHYSICIAN'S HANDBOOK

First Edition

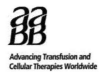

**Advancing Transfusion and
Cellular Therapies Worldwide**

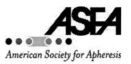

American Society for Apheresis

2005

To purchase books or to inquire about other book services, including chapter reprints and large-quantity sales, please contact our sales department:

- 866.222.2498 (within the United States)
- +1 301.215.6499 (outside the United States)
- +1 301.951.7150 (fax)
- https://portal.aabb.org/apps/marketplace/home.aspx

AABB customer service representatives are available by telephone from 8:30 am to 5:00 pm ET, Monday through Friday, excluding holidays.

Editor
Bruce C. McLeod, MD

Contributing Editors
Kendall Crookston, MD, PhD
Anne Eder, MD, PhD
Karen King, MD
Joseph Kiss, MD
Ravindra Sarode, MD
Jeffrey L. Winters, MD

Handbook Series Editor
Darrell J. Triulzi, MD

Contents

PREFACE

Therapeutic Apheresis: A Physician's Handbook is a joint effort by AABB and the American Society for Apheresis (ASFA). Both organizations saw a need for a succinct guide for clinicians whose patients may benefit from therapeutic apheresis, as well as for physicians and other health-care professionals who carry out apheresis treatments. Indeed, the editors' hope is that, by summarizing information about treatment procedures that may be unfamiliar to members of a patient-care team and information about the illnesses treated that may be unfamiliar to members of an apheresis team, this volume will serve as a kind of convenient bridge between the two groups.

The text is divided into six sections. The introductory section describes apheresis instruments and procedures, including measures that may be necessary to gain access to a patient's circulation. Building on this material it covers hemodynamic, biochemical, and other physiologic changes expected during therapeutic apheresis procedures, as well as the adverse effects that sometimes result from these changes.

The section on cytapheresis covers procedures designed to deplete excess platelets or white cells, mainly from patients with myeloproliferative diseases. In addition, it includes material on photopheresis, a presumably immunomodulatory procedure in which the first step is collection of autologous mononuclear cells. It also covers procedures for collection of autologous hematopoietic progenitor cells intended for subsequent transplantation.

Plasma exchange is the most commonly performed therapeutic apheresis procedure and the section devoted to it is therefore the longest in the book. It describes the application of therapeutic plasma exchange to deplete toxic macromolecules, mainly antibodies, in a wide variety of diseases. The indications for plasma exchange are discussed in separate categories of neurologic, hematologic, renal, rheumatic, and metabolic disorders.

The section on red cell exchange describes variants of the basic procedure as well as special requirements for donor red cells to be transfused in them. It then discusses the role of red cell exchange in preventing and treating complications of sickle cell disease, including the issues surrounding perioperative and obstetric use. Finally, it discusses the use of red cell exchange for severe malaria and babesiosis, diseases caused by protozoa that parasitize red cells.

The section on pediatric apheresis addresses the problems posed when adult-scale instruments are employed to treat smaller pediatric patients. It describes measures that can be taken to overcome these problems and discusses several specific applications that are most commonly encountered in the pediatric patient population.

The final section is on selective depletion. It covers a family of ancillary processes whereby patient plasma separated with an apheresis instrument can be rapidly depleted of a pathogenic component such that the treated plasma can be immediately reinfused to the patient. It includes discussions of specific applications for these processes, such as depletion of low-density lipoproteins and IgG antibodies.

In keeping with the handbook format, the authors and editors have aimed for brevity rather than for exhaustive coverage of any subject. Readers who wish to find more detailed accounts of any material included in this book can explore the bibliographies provided. They may wish to consult chapters on therapeutic apheresis in the AABB Press publication titled *Apheresis: Principles and Practice*, 2nd edition.

The authors and editors wish to extend their appreciation to the leadership of both AABB and ASFA for their support of this project. Special thanks are due to Laurie Munk, Janet McGrath, and Jay Pennington for their enthusiastic assistance in producing this valuable resource.

Bruce C. McLeod, MD
Darrell J. Triulzi, MD
Editors

INTRODUCTION TO THERAPEUTIC APHERESIS: PRINCIPLES, PHYSIOLOGY, AND PATIENT MANAGEMENT

Introduction

The practice of bloodletting is viewed with appropriate skepticism by modern society; however, during the past 50 years the removal of specific parts of circulating blood using apheresis has been shown to be therapeutic—even lifesaving—in many diseases. The term "apheresis" is derived from a Greek word meaning "to take away." The practical definition of therapeutic apheresis is a procedure in which blood is removed from a patient and a portion is removed or otherwise manipulated, with the remainder being returned to the patient. Therapeutic apheresis procedures can be classified as either cell depletions or blood component exchanges. Examples of cell depletion include leukapheresis and plateletpheresis. Blood component exchange includes red cell exchange and plasma exchange.

This chapter 1) examines the scientific principles underlying apheresis instrumentation and procedures as well as how these affect the efficiency of treatment; 2) reviews how these principles influence the medical decision making surrounding apheresis treatment; and 3) describes how physiologic changes associated with apheresis may lead to adverse events, and how these may be anticipated and treated. Subsequent chapters elaborate on therapeutic depletion of cellular components such as platelets and white cells, collection of stem cells, and therapeutic exchange of red cells and plasma. It is only through a remarkable and rapid development of apheresis technology in the last half of the 20th century that most of these procedures are possible.

Apheresis Instruments

Therapeutic apheresis may now be performed effectively using either centrifugation or filtration technology (see Table 1). Centrifugation separates blood elements according to density. Whole blood components include (in order of increasing density) plasma, platelets, lymphocytes and monocytes, granulocytes, and red cells (see also Table 4). Centrifugal instruments operate either by discontinuous or continuous flow. Older discontinuous flow technology alternates between blood removal and reinfusion. Continuous flow devices achieve greater processing efficiency by simultaneously removing and reinfusing processed blood components from the patient. Whole blood is withdrawn by means of an inlet pump. To prevent clotting it is immediately mixed with an anticoagulant solution at a preset ratio, typically 10 to 14 parts whole blood to one part of a citrate anticoagulant such as acid-citrate-dextrose-formula A. Anticoagulated blood enters a centrifugation

Table 1. Examples of Devices Used for Therapeutic Plasma Exchange in the United States

Type	Manufacturer	Device
Centrifugal	Baxter/Fenwal	CS3000
	Fresenius	AS104
	Gambro BCT	Spectra
	Haemonetics	MCS+ (LN9000)
Membrane	Asahi	Plasmaflo
	Gambro BCT	Prisma TPE

chamber where it is separated into component layers. The heavier red cells settle to the radially outward side of the spinning chamber, while the lighter plasma accumulates on the inner side. Outlet tubes at either extreme can remove red cells (and possibly other cellular elements) and plasma, respectively. A third outlet tube may be provided at an intermediate position, if it is desired to remove cellular components of intermediate density (eg, platelets, granulocytes, stem cells). In a component exchange procedure, the unwanted plasma or red cell component is pumped to a waste bag while a replacement pump adds appropriate replacement material to the remaining portions of the patient's blood for return to the patient. In procedures where intermediate density components are removed, the plasma/red cell interface is maintained in a steady position by pumps removing red cells and plasma at flow rates appropriate for the patient's hematocrit.

Membrane filtration technology is conceptually related to hemodialysis and ultrafiltration but employs membranes that are permeable to high-molecular-weight proteins while excluding all cellular elements. Its use is limited to therapeutic plasma exchange (TPE) procedures. Pores with effective sizes ranging from 0.2 to 0.6 micron allow passage of proteins with molecular weights exceeding 500,000 Daltons. Membrane filters in current use have sieving coefficients of 0.9 to 1.0 for most plasma proteins, meaning that the protein composition of the filtrate is nearly identical to plasma, even for very large molecules such as IgM. Workable membrane filters have been fabricated from cellulose diacetate, polyethylene, polypropylene, polyvinylchloride, and other synthetic materials. A typical device features an anticoagulant pump (usually with heparin as the anticoagulant), a blood pump, a replacement fluid pump, and an effluent pump. Blood is directed to the plasma filter by means of the blood pump. Concentrated cellular components excluded by the filter are combined with replacement fluid and returned to the patient.

Studies comparing centrifugal and filtration plasma exchange have found them to be similar with respect to safety and efficiency.[1] Procedures may be performed rapidly with membrane separators because time is not required to set up a centrifugal interface and because heparin anticoagulation avoids the rate-limiting effects of citrate discussed later in this chapter. However, only centrifugation can be used to remove cellular elements; thus, filtration is limited to use in plasma exchange. In addition, systemic heparinization may be disadvantageous, as discussed later in this chapter. In North America, centrifugation techniques are most commonly used for therapeutic apheresis. Filtration-based separation is more commonly used for TPE in many other areas of the world.[2-4]

Principles of Apheresis and Blood Component Exchange

The apheresis practitioner should understand the scientific basis of apheresis as well as the mathematical relationships that govern component exchanges. These principles direct patient management and also aid in anticipation and management of possible side effects. Furthermore, understanding the science behind the disease process and how it relates to the apheresis treatment allows better design of treatment and monitoring of effectiveness.

Modeling the Effects of Therapeutic Plasma Exchange

TPE is both the oldest and most commonly performed therapeutic procedure. It is used here as a prototype to illustrate the mathematical and physiologic principles underlying apheresis. These principles may also be applied to other apheresis procedures.[5]

Therapeutic apheresis is predicated upon two assumptions; namely, that a disease state is causally related to the presence of a substance found in the blood, and that the pathogenic substance in the patient's body can be removed efficiently enough to permit resolution of the illness.[6] Application of these assumptions to modern medical practice led to the treatment of clinical hyperviscosity syndrome in Waldenström's macroglobulinemia during the 1950s.[7]

The extent of constituent removal during TPE depends on the following[6]:

- The volume of plasma removed relative to the patient's total plasma volume.
- The distribution of the substance to be removed between the intravascular and extravascular compartments.
- The rapidity with which that substance equilibrates between compartments.

Figure 1 depicts a simple model of these compartments and the movement of a soluble substance between them during TPE. This model assumes that a newly synthesized soluble substance, such as a plasma protein, preferentially enters the intravascular space. Because synthesis and catabolism are usually balanced, the intravascular mass of a plasma constituent is in a steady state, in equilibrium with that proportion of the substance that resides in the extravascular compartment.[6,8] A one-compartment model is assumed for purposes of TPE; that is, the rate of transfer of the substance between extravascular and intravascular compartments is taken to be low relative to the rate of its removal during the apheresis procedure. In practice, this assumption applies fairly well to IgM, IgG, immune complexes, and other large intravascular molecules such as low-density lipoprotein (LDL).[6,9]

The extent to which TPE depletes a substance from the body is affected by its distribution between intravascular and extravascular compartments.[6,9,10] In the course of a single TPE procedure, removal of IgM and fibrinogen, which are located predominantly in the *intra*vascular compartment, is more complete than removal of IgG, which has a larger *extra*vascular distribution. Lower-molecular-weight compounds that are highly diffusible or subject to active homeostatic regulation in the plasma (such as calcium or potassium) are removed much less efficiently by TPE, in effect behaving as though their intravascular and extravascular masses were exchanged simultaneously.[6,9] The return toward baseline levels of a substance after apheresis is governed by a balance of synthesis, catabolism, and reequilibration between compartments, although the administration of immunosuppressive drugs may affect the contribution of synthesis to the recovery of immunoglobulins after TPE.[6,9]

Figure 2 shows the predicted clearance curve for a substance removed by TPE. An exchange of between 1.3 and 1.5 plasma

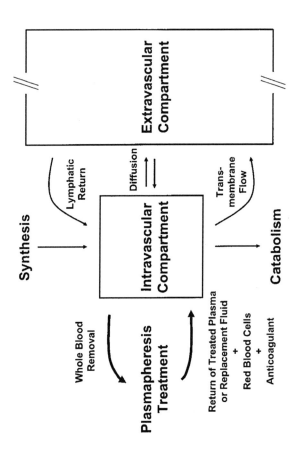

Figure 1. Compartment model of substances removed by therapeutic plasma exchange. Adapted from Weinstein.[6]

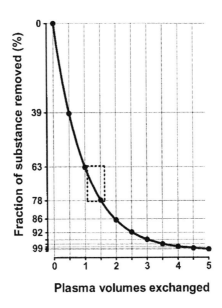

Figure 2. Theoretical curve describing elimination of a substance during apheresis. The equation that describes the removal of a substance of interest in plasma exchange may be written as $y_x = y_0 e^{-x}$ where y_x = final concentration, y_0 = the initial concentration, e = base of natural logarithms, and x = number of patient plasma volumes exchanged (eg, 1.0, 1.3, or 1.5 plasma volumes). The equation assumes that no reequilibration occurs with extravascular stores and that there is no additional synthesis of the substance in question. The dotted line encloses the portion of the graph associated with exchange procedures of 1.0 to 1.5 patient plasma volumes.

volumes would remove about three-fourths of the substance in question. As demonstrated by the graph, increasing the volume of plasma exchanged beyond this gives increasingly diminished returns in terms of substance removal.

In clinical circumstances where the outcome of TPE appears to deviate from prediction according to the one-compartment model (ie, removal of paraproteins), the discrepancy is often attributable to inaccurate estimates of the patient's plasma volume or the concentration of the substance being removed.[6] As Fig 1 suggests, constituent removal during TPE does not always follow the predicted clearance curve.[9] This depends to a large extent on reequilibration with the extravascular compartment. Larger molecules that reside intravascularly (eg, IgM, fibrinogen) generally follow the ideal predictions most closely, while smaller molecules may be depleted much less efficiently than predicted (eg, bilirubin).

Information on constituent clearance during TPE can be helpful in anticipating adverse effects. For example, rapid reequilibration of potassium reduces the apparent efficiency of removal so much that patients rarely become hypokalemic during TPE, even when replacement solutions contain no potassium. Most non-immunoglobulin proteins recover to nearly 100% of baseline within 48 to 72 hours after TPE. A notable exception is fibrinogen, which is discussed in detail below.

Blood and Plasma Volume Calculations

Modern apheresis instruments calculate patient plasma volume automatically using algorithms based on patient height, weight, gender, and hematocrit. Instead of prescribing a specific volume of plasma to be exchanged (eg, 3500 mL), it is sufficient to specify the number of patient "plasma volumes" to be processed (ie, 1.0, 1.3, 1.5). Nevertheless, it is still necessary for a physician to be able to estimate total blood volume (TBV), plasma volume (PV), and red cell volume (RCV) when blood components must be ordered for emergent procedures or to determine whether the extracorporeal blood volume is appropriate in certain procedures or patient populations. TBV, RCV, and PV can be calculated and used 1) to estimate the percentage of the patient's blood and red cells that will be in the extracorporeal circuit during apheresis and 2) to calculate the "apheresis dose." The "dose" may be expressed as the volume of blood to be processed in a therapeutic cytapheresis or the volume of plasma or red cells to be exchanged in a therapeutic component exchange.

8

TBV is between 5.5% and 7.5% of body mass for most adults[11] and may be estimated as 70 mL/kg for males and 65 mL/kg for females (see Table 13). Because TBV increases with muscle mass, this may underestimate TBV for muscular individuals and overestimate it for obese individuals. TBV and hematocrit can be used to estimate plasma volume. The TBV of a 100-kg male would be about 7 L (100 kg × 70 mL/kg = 7000 mL = 7 L). If his hematocrit is 40%, then the RCV would be 2.8 L (0.40 × 7 L) and the remaining 60% of the 7 L would be plasma (0.60 × 7 L = 4.2 L). These relationships underscore that for a given TBV, the volume of plasma treated must be increased as the hematocrit decreases in order to obtain the same intensity of treatment.

To minimize the risk of hypovolemia, the general standard of care is to limit the patient's extracorporeal blood volume to 15% of TBV.[12] All modern continuous flow instruments meet this limit for adults and adolescents. The extracorporeal blood volume or "dead space volume" varies among different instruments, ranging between 150 and 500 mL. Reduction of an adult's blood or red cell volume by this amount is usually tolerated; however, it may be a challenge for a child. Priming the apheresis instrument with a colloid solution or red cells, as described in Chapter 5, may help to prevent intraprocedural hypovolemia and/or the effects of acute anemia in pediatric procedures and in susceptible adult patients. Alternatively, the patient may be given a saline/colloid bolus. Red cell transfusion or priming may be indicated for anemic patients if the extracorporeal red cell volume will exceed 15% of RCV; however, widely accepted criteria for transfusion have not been formulated. The intraprocedure hematocrit (assuming the patient is maintained in an isovolemic state during apheresis) may be more predictive of the patient's tolerance of temporary extracorporeal red cell loss than the extracorporeal percentages. Intraprocedure hematocrit is calculated as [100 × (RCV – extracorporeal red cell volume)/(TBV)]. The extracorporeal red cell volume is equal to the extracorporeal blood volume of the apheresis circuit adjusted for the patient's hematocrit. In the example of the 100-kg male with the hematocrit of 40%, if the extracorporeal volume were 500 mL, then the extracorporeal red cell volume would be 0.2 L (500 mL × 0.40 = 200 mL = 0.2 L). According to the formula above, the intraprocedure hematocrit would fall to 37% [100 × (2.8 L − 0.2 L)/7 L]. Neither asymptomatic adults nor stable pediatric patients generally require red cell transfusions if they have an intraprocedure hematocrit of at least 24% and can tolerate the expanded blood volume that occurs during rinseback.[12] Patients with acute anemia, such as those with thrombotic thrombocytopenic purpura (TTP), may be less tolerant of a lower intraprocedure hematocrit than patients (such as those with chronic renal failure) who have had time to adjust to anemia.

Replacement Fluids

When several liters of plasma are removed in TPE, it is necessary to provide a replacement solution that exerts a colloid osmotic pressure equivalent to that of plasma in order to avoid hypotension and edema. A solution of 4% to 5% human albumin in physiologic saline is a popular choice; solutions of complex carbohydrates such as pentastarch or hetastarch have also been used. Five percent albumin is slightly *hyper*oncotic compared with normal plasma and may cause some expansion of intravascular fluid volume after an exchange procedure. It is pasteurized to prevent transmission of infection. Replacement with fresh frozen plasma (FFP) should be avoided unless it is specifically indicated to treat a disease (eg, TTP), required to correct a plasma factor deficiency (eg, marked hypofibrinogenemia), or needed to prevent dilutional coagulopathy in a patient who is actively bleeding (eg, pulmonary-renal syndrome).

Clinicians familiar with dialysis procedures may request that fluid be "taken off" by TPE, but hypovolemic exchanges should be performed with great caution. Because plasma exchange modulates only intravascular volume, it has very different hemodynamic effects than hemoperfusion or hemodialysis. Severe hypotension can occur with hypovolemic exchanges, even in patients who initially experience volume overload.[5]

Physiology of Therapeutic Apheresis

Anticoagulation and Calcium Regulation

Apheresis procedures require anticoagulation, and citrate has become the anticoagulant of choice in this setting. It anticoagulates by chelating calcium ions and blocking calcium-dependent platelet activation and clotting factor reactions.[5,13,14] The challenge is to strike a balance between adequate anticoagulation and potential toxicity; this requires an understanding of calcium metabolism and the effects of citrate infusion on calcium homeostasis.

Of the total body calcium, 99% is found in bone; a small portion of this can be mobilized rapidly to correct a circulating deficiency. Virtually all of the 1000 mg of nonosseous calcium is extracellular, with the normal plasma concentration being about 10 mg/dL. Roughly 40% of plasma calcium is bound to plasma proteins, primarily albumin, while 13% is complexed to small anions such as lactate, phosphate, and endogenous citrate. The remaining half (47%) of plasma calcium is free, and it is this free (ionized) calcium fraction that participates in coagulation reactions and is chelated by exogenous citrate.[5] The decrease in ionized calcium that results from exogenous citrate infusion also underlies certain adverse events associated with citrate anticoagulants.[13]

Citrate levels observed during apheresis have been reported to range from 17 mg/dL[15] to over 30 mg/dL.[16] During a plateletpheresis procedure this typically leads to a 23% to 33% reduction in ionized calcium.[14,16] Because FFP already contains citrate, using it as a replacement fluid in TPE involves higher rates of citrate infusion than plateletpheresis, but the resultant effects on calcium are similar. Dilution, redistribution, rapid metabolism, and excretion of infused citrate are important factors protecting against profound hypocalcemia. When a calcium-free, citrate-free replacement such as 5% albumin solution is used in TPE, the situation becomes more complex. As noted previously, albumin itself can bind ionized calcium and may contribute to ionized hypocalcemia during TPE.[14,17] Even though much of the citrate infused during TPE is discarded with the separated plasma, an exchange still produces a net loss of calcium.

The net effect of citrate and parathormone levels on plasma calcium is that total calcium decreases most rapidly in the first 15 minutes of a procedure, reaching a 25% decrement by 90 minutes. Intact parathormone rises quickly and then levels off or decreases slightly during the remainder of the procedure.[16] This suggests that, in addition to body weight, TBV, and hematocrit, the rate and duration of citrate infusion may affect the severity of citrate toxicity.[18] Modern apheresis instruments limit both citrate dose and dose rate on the basis of patient blood volume calculations. Therefore, they produce peak citrate and trough ionized calcium levels that are less extreme and have a correspondingly lower incidence of citrate toxicity than in years past. Some centers depend on the increase in parathormone to obviate the need for routine supplementary calcium during therapeutic apheresis procedures. Others routinely use prophylactic calcium replacement in order to prevent citrate reactions (see the section on "citrate-induced hypocalcemia" later in this chapter).[19,20]

Heparin anticoagulation can also be used during an apheresis procedure (although citrate provides a better risk:benefit ratio in most patients); indeed, certain instruments require heparin administration. Adequate anticoagulation is achieved with a plasma heparin concentration of 0.5 to 2.0 IU/mL, which is roughly the same range as (or slightly higher than) that required for therapeutic heparinization for deep vein thrombosis. The implications of using heparin are discussed in greater detail elsewhere.[5]

In summary, moderate hypocalcemia is regularly associated with therapeutic apheresis. It can result from 1) infusion of citrate anticoagulant dispensed by the instrument, 2) infusion of citrate in FFP, and/or 3) infusion of calcium-binding albumin solutions.[17] The degree of hypocalcemia increases with the concentration of citrate used, the rate of infusion, and the duration of the procedure.

Antibody Depletion and Rebound

Antibody levels decline when TPE is performed with albumin replacement. Although increased susceptibility to infection due to decreased circulating antibody might logically be predicted in patients receiving numerous treatments, it is rarely observed. Replacement with plasma or intravenous immune globulin (IVIG) for the purpose of replenishing lost immunoglobulins is not indicated.[21] It has also been proposed that removal of immunoglobulins by TPE stimulates an increase in synthesis that will raise specific antibody titers to levels even higher than baseline (ie, "rebound" phenomenon).[9,22,23] Although not widely accepted by investigators,[24,25] this phenomenon has been the basis of clinical trials of combinations of TPE with immunosuppressive agents for the treatment of various immune-mediated diseases.[26]

Patient Evaluation and Management

Therapeutic apheresis is applied to a broad spectrum of diseases and syndromes that encompass many medical specialties and patients of all ages. Although it has become almost routine clinically, it is an invasive procedure that can have significant physiologic consequences. Not only does the majority of the patient's blood circulate extracorporeally during the procedure, but large amounts of various solutions are returned that can potentially affect electrolytes, oncotic pressure, osmolarity, blood pressure, infection risk, coagulation, temperature control, and general homeostasis. As noted above, the requirement for anticoagulation has a profound effect on several physiologic variables. The procedure itself leads to both hemodynamic and dilutional changes. These physiologic consequences may also result in patient adverse events.

A request for a therapeutic apheresis procedure should result in expert recommendations regarding the role of apheresis in the care of the patient.[11] Table 2 gives an overview of important medical decisions surrounding apheresis treatment.

Patient Assessment

The apheresis physician evaluates all patients who are being considered for therapeutic apheresis. The initial consultation includes

Table 2. Key Medical Decisions in Therapeutic Apheresis

Appropriateness of treatment

- Are there alternative diagnoses?
- What is the disease pathogenesis?
- Is there published experience with therapeutic apheresis for this indication?
- Which modality of therapeutic apheresis is contemplated?
- Is therapeutic apheresis effective?
- Is therapeutic apheresis the primary treatment?
- What is the likelihood that the disease will respond?
- What are the alternatives to therapeutic apheresis?
- Is therapeutic apheresis indicated now?
- What is the risk:benefit ratio of therapeutic apheresis?

Patient assessment and monitoring

- What is the patient's status (renal/fluid balance, cardiovascular, pulmonary, coagulation)?
- Can the patient tolerate the procedure? Give consent?
- Where should the procedure be performed?

Treatment plan and endpoint

- What kind of vascular access is indicated?
- What is the proper "dose" per treatment?
- What are the proper number and frequency of treatments?
- What comorbid conditions might alter the protocol?
- Can the patient tolerate the proposed extracorporeal volume?
- What type of replacement fluids should be prescribed?
- Which baseline laboratory values are most appropriate?
- Will any of the patient's drugs interfere with therapeutic apheresis?
- Will therapeutic apheresis remove or interfere with concurrent medications? Interfere with other treatments? Affect the accuracy of subsequent diagnostic tests?
- Is any premedication needed?
- Will any special monitoring be needed during or after treatment?
- What parameters will be followed to assess efficacy of treatment?
- What is the endpoint of the treatment plan?

a review of the patient's medical history (including medications), physical examination, current laboratory data, and specific markers of disease activity. It is important to confirm the diagnosis, to independently gauge the appropriateness of therapeutic apheresis, and to correctly determine the risks and benefits of the proposed treatment. Coexisting health problems, as well as certain concurrent medications or other treatments, should be considered in planning a course of apheresis therapy. Patients should be reassessed by the apheresis team before each treatment.

Laboratory Evaluation and Monitoring

The frequency of laboratory testing in patients for whom a series of therapeutic apheresis procedures has been prescribed will depend on the disorder being treated, the clinical status of the patient, the type and frequency of the apheresis procedures, and concurrent therapy. A complete blood count, a serum electrolyte panel, and blood urea nitrogen and creatinine levels should be determined for all patients before the first therapeutic apheresis procedure. Serum protein levels, liver function tests, and coagulation screening tests—including fibrinogen—are also useful. Whenever possible, disease-specific markers should be monitored to gauge the efficacy and endpoint of treatment.

Medical Decision Making

Unfortunately, definitive studies do not exist for many of the diseases for which apheresis has been advocated. Therefore, it is necessary to understand the pathogenesis of the treated disease and the principles of apheresis so that an "educated" treatment plan may be designed in the absence of compelling studies and in the face of individual patient complexities. Choices should be based on accumulated clinical experience, an understanding of the pathophysiology of diseases treated, and knowledge of the mechanism of action of therapeutic apheresis in combating these diseases.

In many cases, the decision to initiate therapeutic apheresis is straightforward and can be made by the apheresis physician soon after the diagnosis is confirmed. Conversely, apheresis may be requested under circumstances in which the potential benefit is uncertain. Such requests may arise from an incomplete understanding of disease pathogenesis or from a desire to offer an empiric trial when other therapeutic modalities are exhausted or unavailable. A careful assessment of potential risks and benefits should precede the application of therapeutic apheresis, and caution should be exercised, especially if patients have underlying instabilities that predispose them to untoward events. In such situations, consultative expertise and flexibility on the part of the apheresis physician are essential.

Treatment Plan and Physician Orders

Once the appropriateness of apheresis therapy has been established and the initial patient assessment is complete, the apheresis physician develops a treatment plan and appropriate orders. The physician's orders and treatment plan should address the concerns listed in Table 2. The plan should be updated as needed, based on patient reevaluation. Diseases that are not self-limited may require repeat courses of apheresis, depending on the kinetics of constituent resynthesis (eg, IgG with an approximate 21-day half-life vs IgM with a 5- to 6-day half-life) and the ability of pharmaceutical intervention to slow synthesis and/or control symptoms after the initial course.[6]

Specific patient consent for therapeutic apheresis procedures is required, ensuring communication of the risks and anticipated benefits with the patient or legal designee. This includes discussion of alternatives to apheresis, possible outcomes (with and without apheresis), and a risk:benefit ratio assessment tailored to the individual patient.

Vascular Access

Adequate blood flow to and from the machine must be established to perform any type of apheresis procedure. The requisite vascular access may be obtained via peripheral veins, central veins, or a combination of the two. Generally, the flow rate should allow the procedure to be completed in less than 3 hours unless the procedure is a large-volume leukapheresis. The blood flow rate for an adult procedure is usually between 60 and 120 mL/minute, depending on the procedure being performed and the type of replacement fluid; for small children it will need to be lower. The major factors limiting flow rate are the type of vascular access and the patient's ability to tolerate citrate, which is usually related to TBV.

To evaluate the antecubital veins, a tourniquet or blood pressure cuff inflated to the patient's diastolic pressure should be applied 2 to 3 inches above the elbow. The veins should increase in size and have a spongy feel when palpated. Good muscle tone in the arms helps to maintain blood flow; consequently, patients with peripheral neuropathies, who cannot forcefully contract their arm muscles to make a tight fist, may be unable to maintain adequate flow with peripheral access. To avoid infection, the skin preparation before venipuncture should be the same as for a blood donation procedure. If desired, the skin may be anesthetized with intradermal lidocaine, topical ethyl chloride, or topical EMLA cream (lidocaine 2.5% and prilocaine 2.5%). Thin-walled steel needles are recommended for the draw line because they have the smallest possible outer diameter for the gauge size. A needle with a back eye (opening on the opposite side of the bevel) may allow a higher maximum flow. Peripheral intravenous (IV) catheters tend to collapse when used as draw lines but can make excellent return lines. A 17- to 18-gauge line is recommended for return flows above 80 mL/minute, while a 19-gauge line will suffice for return flows below 70 mL/minute.[12] Return lines in lower-arm or hand veins allow some arm movement and save the antecubital veins for future draw sites.

If peripheral access is not possible, insertion of an artificial access device may be indicated. However, a central venous catheter (CVC) represents the single greatest risk factor for adverse events associated with therapeutic apheresis,[27] and it should be avoided whenever possible.[28] CVCs are more likely to be needed in patients who require frequent procedures over an extended period (eg, TTP, pulmonary-renal syndrome) or have decreased muscle tone and/or autonomic instability (eg, myasthenic crisis, acute Guillain-Barré syndrome).[29,30] Temporary percutaneous

CVCs and semipermanent tunneled CVCs designed for apheresis or dialysis can provide adequate blood flow. The choice between them is dictated by clinical factors, in particular the expected duration of apheresis therapy and/or other therapies requiring such a device. A silver-impregnated cuff attached to the catheter at the time of insertion has been shown to reduce infection.[12] Peripherally inserted central venous catheters (PICC lines), standard implantable ports (Port-a-Cath), and the standard (nondialysis) double/triple-lumen catheters rarely provide flow rates adequate for adults.

Recirculation

Recirculation (removal of fluid that has just been returned) is a risk with dual-lumen catheters. It can be a major problem when there is a downstream blockage near the catheter tip. In such cases, the same blood may be recycled continually. If, at the start of the procedure, the return saline is observed entering the draw line (clear or dilute input line), or if a plasma-red cell interface fails to develop in the centrifugal module, recirculation is the most likely explanation. In some instances, a fibrinolytic agent such as tissue plasminogen activator (tPA) may be of benefit, but usually the catheter must be replaced. Some degree of recirculation may occur when the ports of a CVC are reversed (ie, the proximal port is used for return and the distal port is used for draw). In general, however, the intravascular blood flow rate past the CVC tip is high enough relative to flow rates through the CVC that recirculation is minimal.

Paraprotein Removal

Removal of monoclonal immunoglobulins from patients with multiple myeloma, Waldenström's macroglobulinemia, and other paraproteinemic states may seem less than optimally efficient.[6] This is most likely a result of the plasma volume expansion expected in such patients, which makes standard formulas underestimate PV and intravascular protein load.

Coagulation Status

When plasma is exchanged for a nonplasma replacement solution, coagulopathy resulting from dilution of coagulation factors is a potential problem. The prothrombin time and activated partial thromboplastin time rise and fibrinogen levels fall to an extent related to the intensity of the exchange.[6] Despite these hemostatic alterations, hemorrhagic complications of dilutional coagulopathy are seldom encountered unless a patient is hemostatically compromised before treatment.[31] Routine supplementation of replacement fluids with FFP or other sources of clotting factors is not recommended for nonbleeding patients whose baseline coagulation is normal.[9] As mentioned above, redistribution and ongoing synthesis raise levels of most coagulation factors rapidly in the hours following an exchange. Fibrinogen is usually replaced more slowly, although the production of this acute phase protein varies greatly among patients. Fibrinogen levels may decrease somewhat below 100 mg/dL if several procedures are performed on consecutive days. A level near 100 mg/mL is generally sufficient for hemostasis unless the individual has another hemostatic challenge; however, if fibrinogen levels fall much below 100 mg/dL, many physicians increase the interval between procedures or supplement fibrinogen during the last part of the procedure to avoid a bleeding diathesis.[13] FFP is the preferred source of fibrinogen and supplies other coagulation factors as well, but it is seldom required if TPE is performed at intervals of 72 hours or greater.

Regardless of the replacement fluid used, coagulation testing during or in the hours after an apheresis treatment should be avoided, as the tests may be artifactually prolonged by the procedure. Waiting until the next morning to draw blood for coagulation studies will give a better picture of underlying coagulation status. A fibrinogen level is always useful in evaluating prolonged coagulation tests in an apheresis patient, as clotting times may be lengthened artificially due to lack of fibrinogen substrate rather than a generalized coagulopathy. Also, in a patient with unexpectedly prolonged clotting times, it is not infrequently discovered that the specimen was drawn through a heparin-anticoagulated catheter.

Alkalosis

Metabolism of citrate consumes hydrogen ions and produces bicarbonate ions. In patients with renal disease whose maximal bicarbonate excretion rate is reduced, infusion of citrate often leads to metabolic alkalosis.[32] This is most often seen with TPE when the replacement fluid is FFP.[33,34] Alkalosis may make patients more susceptible to adverse consequences of hypocalcemia and could slow citrate metabolism.[33] Alkalosis induced by a citrate load from an apheresis procedure will resolve with time or dialysis.

Hemodynamic Changes

Another major category of physiologic responses to therapeutic apheresis is fluid shifts that occur as whole blood is removed, one or another component is retained, and the remaining components are returned, with or without replacement solution. Resultant changes in intravascular volume can induce hemodynamic alterations. Fluid overload may be a problem for patients with cardiac or renal impairment. In other situations, hypovolemia may be a concern. There is a general sense that hemodynamic changes are more common with intermittent flow centrifugation than with continuous flow procedures. This probably relates to the greater extracorporeal volume associated with earlier models of intermittent flow machines.

Different procedures may also produce differing hemodynamic effects. In simple plateletpheresis, a relatively small net volume deficit (approximately 300 mL plasma) develops gradually over 60 to 100 minutes. In leukapheresis, a somewhat larger volume of plasma may be removed along with the leukocytes; however, infusion of a sedimenting agent with volume-expanding properties tends to offset this. Similarly, hematopoietic stem cell apheresis may remove a substantial amount of plasma.

Dilutional Effects

TPE with albumin replacement has the greatest potential for volume shifts and dilutional effects. In addition to coagulation factors mentioned above, TPE can remove pharmacologic agents. The quantity of a drug that is removed depends on its volume of distribution (intravascular vs other), its half-life in the circulation, and whether it is administered immediately before or during apheresis. For example, only about 1% of prednisone is removed by TPE,[35] while agents that remain in the circulation (eg, therapeutic antibodies) will be removed in proportion to the amount of plasma processed. TPE may also influence drug levels indirectly by reducing plasma levels of proteins that bind and transport drugs and/or of enzymes that metabolize them.[5]

Cellular Loss

As large volumes of donor or patient blood circulate through an apheresis device, blood cells are intentionally or incidentally removed. The effects of single apheresis procedures have been studied extensively, especially in the setting of platelet donation. The thrust of these studies is that individual apheresis procedures produce only modest decreases in circulating blood cell counts, which are not associated with any immediate toxicity.[5] Reductions in platelet count resulting from adherence to the surfaces of the apheresis circuit are usually modest and levels quickly return to baseline. However, in a severely thrombocytopenic patient, this loss may mask the beginning of platelet recovery. Similarly, the small amount of red cells lost in the apheresis circuit may be noticed in an anemic patient with meager production capacity who is undergoing multiple procedures. Although generally well tolerated, large-volume leukapheresis for stem cell collections in patients often results in a decline in hematocrit and platelet count.

Plasma Protein Interactions

Plasma contains enzymes that can theoretically be activated during apheresis by contact with foreign surfaces. Activation of the clotting cascade is prevented by the anticoagulant, but other systems have also been of concern. Activation of enzymes in the kinin system has been noted in association with protein A immunoadsorption columns and selective depletion columns for LDL removal.[36] Angiotensin-converting enzyme (ACE) inhibitors are contraindicated in patients receiving such therapeutic procedures because they may decrease a patient's ability to inactivate bradykinin, which can lead to flushing, hypotension, and/or respiratory distress.

Adverse Events During Apheresis

Unfortunately, even with the most careful planning and monitoring, adverse reactions may occur during therapeutic apheresis. Physiologic changes expected with apheresis can also sometimes become extreme enough to qualify as adverse effects. The onset of symptoms may be gradual or sudden. The most important aspect in the treatment of these complications is the correct diagnosis of the underlying cause.

Overall Incidence

The rate of adverse events during therapeutic apheresis is 4% to 5%, with the risk being slightly higher during the first procedure, and varying considerably based on the type of procedure.[24] Table 3 lists the frequency of common adverse events from a survey of 3429 therapeutic procedures carried out at 18 US institutions.[2] Expected physiologic consequences of apheresis, such as peripheral and perioral paresthesias and mild light-headedness, were not included as adverse events. Among the most commonly performed procedures, the risk was higher for procedures involving allogeneic red cell or plasma transfusion, and lower for hematopoietic stem cell collection.[5]

Morbidity and mortality related to therapeutic procedures are greater in acutely ill patients treated in a hospital setting than in "routine" patients treated in an outpatient setting. No fatalities were attributed to apheresis during 20,485 procedures reported from the Swedish registry.[3] The French apheresis registry calcu-

Table 3. Most Common Adverse Events in Therapeutic Apheresis[2]

Event/Reaction	Rate (%)
Overall adverse event	4.8
First-time procedure	6.9
Repeat procedure	4.3
Procedure-specific reaction	
Red cell exchange	10.3
Plasma exchange (plasma replacement)	7.8
Leukapheresis	5.7
Plasma exchange (no plasma)	3.4
Autologous stem cell collection	1.7
Type of reaction	
Transfusion reactions	1.6
Citrate-related nausea and/or vomiting	1.2
Hypotension	1.0
Vasovagal nausea and/or vomiting	0.5
Pallor and/or diaphoresis	0.5
Tachycardia	0.4
Respiratory distress	0.3
Tetany or seizure	0.2
Chills or rigors	0.2

lated an overall mortality between 1 in 10,000 and 2 in 10,000.[2] A patient death during an apheresis series is most often attributed to the underlying disease and is rarely directly related to the procedure.[1,37]

Citrate-Induced Hypocalcemia

Transient hypocalcemia associated with apheresis is usually well-tolerated; nevertheless, certain physiologic consequences may be encountered. Decreases in ionized calcium can increase the excitability of nerve cell membranes, allowing spontaneous depolarization. This most often manifests in adults as perioral and/or peripheral paresthesias. Less frequently, patients may experience dysgeusia (loss of or altered taste), nausea, and/or light-headedness. Shivering, twitching, and tremors are rare but have also been reported.[15,37] Some patients may have unusual disease-specific citrate effects, such as intraprocedural worsening of myasthenic weakness.[38] The threshold for developing clinical features of hypocalcemia reflects the absolute ionized calcium level and also the rate of decrease. Serum pH, the presence of sedatives, and concomitant decreases in magnesium, potassium, and/or sodium may also affect the threshold.[5]

Severe hypocalcemia may cause continuous muscle contractions, initially in the form of involuntary carpopedal spasm (adduction of thumbs; extension of interphalangeal joints; and flexion of metacarpophalangeal, wrist, and elbow joints). If hypocalcemia is not corrected, symptoms can progress to frank tetany with spasms in other muscle groups, including life-threatening laryngospasm. Grand mal seizures have also been reported. Appropriate physical examination may reveal evidence of neuromuscular irritability before the onset of spontaneous muscle spasms. Chvostek's sign is positive with marked facial twitching when the facial nerve is tapped, and Trousseau's sign is positive when carpal spasm is seen with ≤3 minutes of cuff-induced arm ischemia. The clinician should remember that these symptoms and signs can also be seen with alkalosis, especially respiratory alkalosis due to hyperventilation.[39] Reductions of ionized calcium seen in apheresis can also lengthen the plateau phase of myocardial depolarization, which leads to prolongation of the QT interval in the electrocardiogram (EKG).

Management of citrate overload during apheresis is straightforward in most cases. Communicative subjects should be asked to report if tingling or numbness is noted. They should also be questioned about paresthesias periodically during the procedure.

In a noncommunicative patient, an EKG pattern may be monitored, if necessary. QT prolongation is difficult to quantify and interpret on a monitor screen, but new arrhythmias and QRS widening are detectable entities that may be signs of clinically significant reductions in ionized calcium.[33] When available, STAT ionized calcium levels may be drawn before and during procedures on patients who experience significant symptoms of hypocalcemia. This will enable the clinician to correlate patient signs and symptoms with the calcium level, to monitor response to calcium infusion, and to tailor future treatment to the specific patient. If paresthesias are bothersome, either the total blood flow rate or the rate at which anticoagulant is added to whole blood in the instrument should be reduced. If tingling becomes severe or is associated with nausea, the procedure can be interrupted until symptoms subside and then resumed with a lower citrate flow rate. Oral calcium supplementation, either before or during apheresis, may be useful in preventing mild reactions.[40] A controlled study is still needed to assess the benefit of prophylactic calcium administration during therapeutic apheresis.

If significant paresthesias, carpopedal spasm, tetany, or EKG changes develop, parenteral calcium supplementation should be considered. Ten percent calcium gluconate may be administered as an IV bolus (5-10 mL infused over 10 to 15 minutes).[5,41] Ten percent calcium chloride may also be infused cautiously; however, calcium gluconate is considered a safer alternative by some, as it is only one-third as potent with respect to calcium ions.[14] In certain centers, supplemental calcium is routinely administered intravenously during therapeutic apheresis in an effort to avoid symptoms of hypocalcemia. Physiologic quantities of calcium may be provided as scheduled IV boluses or added to 5% albumin infused during TPE (10 mL of 10% calcium gluconate per liter of replacement fluid). Calcium should not be added directly to FFP because it will activate clotting factors. For procedures using FFP replacement or for stem cell collections, a calcium infusion may be run in a separate IV line.[19,20]

If 10% calcium chloride is used to treat hypocalcemia instead of 10% calcium gluconate, only one-third the volume should be used because it contains three times more calcium ions. Apheresis programs should consider a policy of using only one calcium preparation routinely to avoid confusion and potential lethal overdose.

Vasovagal Reactions

Vasovagal reactions, the most common reactions seen with whole blood donation, are also observed during and after apheresis.[42] They generally manifest as pallor and diaphoresis, with associated hypotension and bradycardia. In a full-blown attack, the following progression is often observed: 1) pallor and sweating begin, with the skin turning cold; 2) the pulse slows strikingly, sometimes to as low as 30 beats per minute; and 3) the blood pressure falls. More severe vasovagal reactions may include nausea, vomiting, and/or syncope, with involuntary defecation and/or convulsions. All these phenomena have been related to imbalances in autonomic tone. The slow pulse rate is the most useful sign in differentiating vasovagal effects from hypovolemia. Attacks are best treated by maintaining the patient in a supine position with the head below the legs (Trendelenberg position). The apheresis procedure should be halted until the reaction is reversed.

Problems Related to Vascular Access

Adverse effects related to vascular access are a frequent concern. Hematoma, venous sclerosis, and thrombosis can complicate percutaneous needle puncture. Hemorrhage and/or pneumothorax may complicate CVC insertion, while thrombosis and infection are the most frequently observed complications of prolonged central venous access. During a dressing change, the site should be cleaned and observed for signs of infection such as redness, swelling, drainage, and foul odor. If an infection is suspected, the CVC should be removed and cultured, and a different site should be used for access. The cause of a CVC flow problem may be difficult to determine, although patient repositioning will sometimes improve flow. A common situation is that the CVC can be flushed without resistance but does not yield blood return; this may be the result of kinking, poor positioning, intralumenal clots, or venous thrombosis. Blocked CVCs can sometimes be cleared with a fibrinolytic agent such as tPA.[12]

Allergic Reactions

Allergic reactions are usually associated with replacement regimens that include blood components, but they can also be caused by medications, hydroxyethyl starch, or sterilization of disposable tubing with ethylene oxide. Symptoms may include hives, dyspnea, wheezing, hypotension, tachycardia, facial swelling or flushing, and burning eyes. Mild allergic reactions can be treated initially with 25 to 50 mg of diphenhydramine administered "IV push." For symptoms of anaphylaxis, 0.3 to 0.5 mL of epinephrine, 1:1000 (1 mg/mL), may be given subcutaneously or intramuscularly in an adult.[12,43] For a child between 6 and 12 years of age, 0.25 mL has been recommended. The epinephrine dose may be repeated in 10 to 15 minutes if no response is seen. The patient's heart rate should be closely monitored. Intravenous epinephrine may be used cautiously for severe anaphylaxis; however, a dilution is required. One adult protocol suggests dilution of 0.1 mL of a 1:1000 (1 mg/mL) epinephrine solution into 10 mL saline and very careful infusion of the 10-mL dose intravenously over 5 to 10 minutes.[12,43] Methylprednisolone (Solumedrol, Upjohn, Don Mills, Ontario, Canada), 100 mg given intravenously, can also be administered.[12] A specific protocol for treatment of anaphylaxis should be prepared in advance under direction of the apheresis physician.

Drug Interactions

Drugs used to treat certain conditions may block the natural physiologic response to changes in intravascular volume. For example, beta blockers may prevent an increase in heart rate in response to hypotension, and calcium channel blockers and nitroglycerin paste may prevent vasoconstriction in response to volume shifts. ACE inhibitors may increase the risk of allergic/anaphylactoid reactions. It is important for a physician to evaluate the interplay between the patient's medications and illness and the potential interactions with the selected apheresis treatment.[5]

Miscellaneous Reactions

Several other rare reactions are mentioned in passing here.[2,5,13] Potential mechanical problems include hemolysis, clotting, and air embolism. Granulocyte colony-stimulating factor (filgrastim) stimulation of stem cell donors may lead to significant bone pain in some donors. Another potential problem is the removal of cholinesterase, which would increase a subsequent anesthesia risk if urgent surgery were required. Delayed complications include hemorrhage, thrombosis, infection related to access lines or blood components, anemia, and protein depletion.

Conclusion

In summary, patient management during therapeutic apheresis is based on knowledge of basic apheresis principles and the mathematics involved. Combined with an understanding of the disease process, this allows planning of treatments and anticipation of side effects. Therefore, a solid scientific understanding, both of apheresis and of the pathophysiology of the disease to be treated, is important for the apheresis physician. Therapeutic apheresis procedures may lead to major physiologic changes, including hypocalcemia due to citrate infusion, hemodynamic changes associated with fluid shifts, and depletion of cellular and plasma constituents. Because a greater understanding of the physiology of apheresis has guided continued improvements in technology, the potential for untoward effects has been minimized so that procedures may usually be performed without adverse events.

References

1. Gurland HJ, Lysaght MJ, Samtleben W, Schmidt B. A comparison of centrifugal and membrane-based apheresis formats. Int J Artif Organs 1984;7:35-8.

2. McLeod BC, Sniecinski I, Ciavarella D, et al. Frequency of immediate adverse effects associated with therapeutic apheresis. Transfusion 1999;39:282-8.

3. Korach JM, Petitpas D, Poiron L, et al. 14 years of therapeutic plasma exchange in France. Transfus Apheresis Sci 2001;25:73-7.

4. Norda R, Stegmayr BG. Therapeutic apheresis in Sweden: Update of epidemiology and adverse events. Transfus Apheresis Sci 2003;29:159-66.

5. Crookston KP, Simon TL. Physiology of apheresis. In: McLeod BC, Price TH, Weinstein R, eds. Apheresis: Principles and practice. 2nd ed. Bethesda, MD: AABB Press, 2003:71-93.

6. Weinstein R. Basic principles of therapeutic blood exchange. In: McLeod BC, Price TH, Weinstein R, eds. Apheresis: Principles and practice. 2nd ed. Bethesda, MD: AABB Press, 2003:295-320.

7. Reynolds WA. Late report of the first case of plasmapheresis for Waldenström's macroglobulinemia. JAMA 1981;245:606-7.

8. Kellogg RM, Hester JP. Kinetics modeling of plasma exchange: Intra- and post-plasma exchange. J Clin Apheresis 1988;4:183-7.

9. Orlin JB, Berkman EM. Partial plasma exchange using albumin replacement: Removal and recovery of normal plasma constituents. Blood 1980;56:1055-9.

10. Morgenthaler JJ, Nydegger UE. Synthesis, distribution and catabolism of human plasma proteins in plasma exchange. Int J Artif Organs 1984;7:27-34.

11. Gilcher RO. Apheresis: Principles and technology of hemapheresis. In: Simon TL, Dzik WH, Snyder EL, et al, eds. Rossi's principles of transfusion medicine. 3rd ed. Philadelphia: Lippincott, Williams & Wilkins, 2002:648-61.

12. Jones HG, Bandarenko N. Management of the therapeutic apheresis patient. In: McLeod BC, Price TH, Weinstein R, eds. Apheresis: Principles and practice. 2nd ed. Bethesda, MD: AABB Press, 2003:253-82.

29

13. Strauss RG, McLeod BC. Complications of therapeutic apheresis. In: Popovsky MA, ed. Transfusion reactions. 2nd ed. Bethesda, MD: AABB Press, 2001:315-38.
14. Hester JP, Ayyar R. Anticoagulation and electrolytes. J Clin Apheresis 1984;2:41-51.
15. Szymanski IO. Ionized calcium during plateletpheresis. Transfusion 1978;18:701-8.
16. Bolan CD, Greer SE, Cecco SA, et al. Comprehensive analysis of citrate effects during plateletpheresis in normal donors. Transfusion 2001;41:1165-71.
17. Weinstein R. Hypocalcemic toxicity and atypical reactions in therapeutic plasma exchange. J Clin Apheresis 2001;16: 210-1.
18. Hester JP, McCullough J, Mishler JM, Szymanski IO. Dosage regimens for citrate anticoagulants. J Clin Apheresis 1983;1:149-57.
19. Korach JM, Berger P, Giraud C, et al. Role of replacement fluids in the immediate complications of plasma exchange. Intensive Care Med 1998;24:452-8.
20. Bolan CD, Cecco SA, Wesley RA, et al. Controlled study of citrate effects and response to IV calcium administration during allogeneic peripheral blood progenitor cell donation. Transfusion 2002;42:935-46.
21. Schmaldienst S, Mullner M, Goldammer A, et al. Intravenous immunoglobulin application following immunoadsorption: Benefit or risk in patients with autoimmune diseases? Rheumatology (Oxford) 2001;40:513-21.
22. Dau PC. Immunologic rebound. J Clin Apheresis 1995; 10:210-7.
23. Derksen RH, Schuurman HJ, Gmelig Meyling FH, et al. Rebound and overshoot after plasma exchange in humans. J Lab Clin Med 1984;104:35-43.
24. Goldammer A, Derfler K, Herkner K, et al. Influence of plasma immunoglobulin level on antibody synthesis. Blood 2002;100:353-5.
25. Junghans RP. IgG biosynthesis: No "immunoregulatory feedback." Blood 1997;90:3815-8.
26. Blume G, Pestronk A, Goodnough LT. Anti-MAG antibody-associated polyneuropathies: Improvement follow-

ing immunotherapy with monthly plasma exchange and IV cyclophosphamide. Neurology 1995;45:1577-80.

27. Spindler JS. Subclavian vein catheterization for apheresis access. J Clin Apheresis 1983;1:202-5.

28. Noseworthy JH, Shumak KH, Vandervoort MK. Long-term use of antecubital veins for plasma exchange. Transfusion 1989;29:610-3.

29. Rizvi MA, Vesely SK, George JN, et al. Complications of plasma exchange in 71 consecutive patients treated for clinically suspected thrombotic thrombocytopenic purpura-hemolytic-uremic syndrome. Transfusion 2000;40:896-901.

30. Annane D, Baudrie V, Blanc AS, et al. Short-term variability of blood pressure and heart rate in Guillain-Barré syndrome without respiratory failure. Clin Sci (Lond) 1999;96:613-21.

31. Flaum MA, Cuneo RA, Appelbaum FR, et al. The hemostatic imbalance of plasma-exchange transfusion. Blood 1979;54:694-702.

32. Kelleher SP, Schulman G. Severe metabolic alkalosis complicating regional citrate hemodialysis. Am J Kidney Dis 1987;9:235-6.

33. Dzik WH, Kirkley SA. Citrate toxicity during massive blood transfusion. Transfus Med Rev 1988;2:76-94.

34. Pearl RG, Rosenthal MH. Metabolic alkalosis due to plasmapheresis. Am J Med 1985;79:391-3.

35. Stigelman WH Jr, Henry DH, Talbert RL, Townsend RJ. Removal of prednisone and prednisolone by plasma exchange. Clin Pharm 1984;3:402-7.

36. Owen HG, Brecher ME. Atypical reactions associated with use of angiotensin-converting enzyme inhibitors and apheresis. Transfusion 1994;34:891-4.

37. Olson PR, Cox C, McCullough J. Laboratory and clinical effects of the infusion of ACD solution during platelet-pheresis. Vox Sang 1977;33:79-87.

38. Wirguin I, Brenner T, Shinar E, Argov Z. Citrate-induced impairment of neuromuscular transmission in human and experimental autoimmune myasthenia gravis. Ann Neurol 1990;27:328-30.

39. Bruder JM, Guise TA, Mundy GR. Mineral metabolism. In: Felig P, Frohman LA, eds. Endocrinology and metabolism. New York: McGraw-Hill, 2001:1079-177.
40. Kishimoto M, Ohto H, Shikama Y, et al. Treatment for the decline of ionized calcium levels during peripheral blood progenitor cell harvesting. Transfusion 2002;42:1340-7.
41. Couriel D, Weinstein R. Complications of therapeutic plasma exchange: A recent assessment. J Clin Apheresis 1994;9:1-5.
42. McLeod BC, Sniecinski I, Ciavarella D, et al. Frequency of immediate adverse effects associated with apheresis donation. Transfusion 1998;38:938-43.
43. Lieberman P. Use of epinephrine in the treatment of anaphylaxis. Curr Opin Allergy Clin Immunol 2003;3: 313-8.

CYTAPHERESIS

Introduction

The purpose of a cytapheresis procedure is to deplete or collect a component of the buffy coat—ie, a blood cell whose density is intermediate between red cells and plasma (Table 4). Such procedures were the original purpose for which all families of centrifugal apheresis instruments were intended; indeed, these instruments are often called "blood cell separators."

By adjusting variables such as the centrifugal force applied, the geometry of the separation chamber or, for intermittent collection techniques, the timing of collection events, it is possible to design procedures that emphasize collection of either platelets or mononuclear cells (MNCs or white cells). The addition of a rouleaux-promoting agent such as hydroxyethyl starch (HES) to whole blood entering the centrifuge will accelerate sedimentation of red cells in the centrifugal field. This improves the separation of red cells from granulocytes [polymorphonuclear cells (PMNs)], whose density exceeds that of MNCs and is very close to that of the youngest red cells; thus, collection of PMNs by an apheresis instrument is enhanced.[2]

This chapter covers all types of cytapheresis procedures used to treat patients, although, strictly speaking, the term "therapeutic cytapheresis" might be reserved for procedures intended to deplete an overabundant and/or abnormal cellular component. Other cytapheresis procedures might be better characterized as autologous donations, in that the expected benefit will not accrue until the collected cells are reinfused at some future time. Reinfusion of unmanipulated peripheral blood progenitor cells, for example, may restore hematopoiesis, while reinfusion of cells

Table 4. Density of Blood Components

Component	Specific Gravity
Plasma	1.025-1.029
Platelets	1.040
Lymphocytes	1.050-1.061
Monocytes	1.065-1.070
Granulocytes	1.087-1.092
Red cells	1.093-1.096

that have been materially altered ex vivo may confer enhanced immunity or correct a genetic defect.

The extent to which the blood concentration of a targeted cell will be reduced by a therapeutic cytapheresis procedure is difficult to predict. Formulas based on blood volume, initial cell concentration, and volume processed tend to give inaccurate estimates because 1) blood volume may be underestimated by standard nomograms, 2) additional cells may be mobilized from marrow or an enlarged spleen during a procedure, and/or 3) the sedimentation behavior of abnormal cells may differ from expectations.[2] For these reasons it is unwise to prescribe a specific volume to be processed in a therapeutic cytapheresis procedure. Rather, it is preferable to monitor the blood cell count of interest during a procedure and stop only when a meaningful reduction has been achieved (eg, 30%-50%).

Therapeutic Plateletpheresis

A supranormal platelet count may occur in three settings. Rare familial cases may be caused by excess thrombopoietin production. Reactive thrombocytosis can develop in response to a variety of primary events including splenectomy, iron deficiency, chronic inflammation, and malignancy. Finally, an elevated platelet count may be seen in clonal myeloproliferative disorders such as chronic myelogenous leukemia. When thrombocytosis is the only manifestation of an abnormal clone, the disorder is called essential thrombocythemia. Symptoms arising from an elevated platelet count are seen only in patients who have a myeloproliferative disorder.[3,4]

Many patients with an elevated platelet count remain asymptomatic indefinitely; however, both thrombosis and hemorrhage are noted with increased frequency in the subset with myeloproliferative disorders. Thrombosis may be venous (eg, deep vein thrombosis, Budd-Chiari syndrome) or arterial (eg, erythromelalgia, stroke). Bleeding may be the result of a platelet function defect or aspirin given for prophylaxis against thrombosis. An age greater than 60 years, a preexisting cardiovascular disease, or a history of thrombosis confers an increased risk for clinical events, the degree of which seems to correlate roughly with the platelet count. By contrast, in younger patients without cardiovascular disease, the risk of clinical events seems to be independent of platelet count; ie, problems may develop at a platelet count of 500,000/μL in some patients, yet others may remain asymptomatic for years with platelet counts exceeding 1,000,000/μL.[3,4]

There is little hard evidence to guide decisions about therapy for thrombocytosis. One trial in high-risk patients showed a lower incidence of clinical events when the platelet count was maintained below 600,000/μL,[5] but there are no comparable data for other patient groups. Pharmacologic therapy with hydroxyurea or anagrelide will lower the platelet count eventually in most cases. Therapeutic plateletpheresis is generally reserved for patients with acute, serious thrombotic or hemorrhagic events or for high-risk patients who present with very high platelet counts. Thrombocytosis in such circumstances has been rated a Category I (standard practice) indication for therapeutic plateletpheresis by the American Society for Apheresis (ASFA)[6] and AABB[7] (Table 5). A single plateletpheresis will lower the platelet count rapidly, and follow-up procedures can maintain a lower level until pharmacologic therapy takes effect.[2,3]

Table 5. ASFA and AABB Indication Categories for Therapeutic Cell Depletion[6,7]

Disease	Procedure	ASFA/AABB Category
Thrombocytosis	Plateletpheresis	I
Hyperleukocytosis	Leukapheresis	I
Rheumatoid arthritis	Lymphoplasmapheresis	II
Progressive multiple sclerosis	Leukapheresis	III
Inclusion body myositis	Leukapheresis	IV
Polymyositis	Leukapheresis	IV
Dermatomyositis	Leukapheresis	IV
Heart transplant rejection	Photopheresis	III
Cutaneous T-cell lymphoma	Photopheresis	I
	Leukapheresis	III

Category I = standard acceptable therapy; Category II = available evidence suggests efficacy; Category III = available evidence is inconclusive; Category IV = ineffective in controlled trials.

Therapeutic plateletpheresis can be performed with any centrifugal apheresis instrument. Anticoagulation, centrifuge speed, and separatory chamber configuration are generally the same as those used for a platelet donation; however, a higher flow rate in the component removal line may be desirable in an instrument so equipped.[2] As mentioned above, it is difficult to predict the platelet count decrement based solely on the volume of blood processed in such a procedure. Therefore, STAT intraprocedural platelet counts are necessary to ensure that a given decrement (eg, a 50% decline) is achieved before a procedure is discontinued.

Therapeutic Leukapheresis

Therapeutic depletion of nonmalignant lymphocytes, with or without simultaneous plasma exchange, has been reported in several autoimmune disorders. Among these, rheumatoid arthritis, progressive multiple sclerosis, inclusion body myositis, polymyositis, and dermatomyositis have been assigned ASFA/AABB indication categories (Table 5)[6,7]; however, lymphocyte depletion by leukapheresis has not become an accepted therapy in any autoimmune disease. Leukapheresis for removal of malignant lymphocytes in Sezary syndrome associated with cutaneous T-cell lymphoma (CTCL), a Category III indication (Table 5),[6,7] has been largely superseded by photopheresis, as discussed below. Thus the great majority of therapeutic leukapheresis procedures are carried out to treat hyperleukocytosis occurring in association with leukemia.

Rationale

The clinical manifestations attributed to an elevated white cell count in patients with leukemia can be grouped into three categories: leukostasis, tumor lysis syndrome, and early mortality. Although they are not necessarily mutually exclusive, it is useful to keep all three in mind when considering the potential benefits of therapeutic leukapheresis.

Clinically, leukostasis refers to evidence of organ dysfunction due to microvascular obstruction and consequent patchy ischemia. Neurologic abnormalities and pulmonary insufficiency are the most common examples in acute leukemia, while priapism is an additional possible complication in chronic myelogenous leukemia (CML). The pathologic correlate of these symptoms is believed to be small-vessel occlusion by masses of leukemic cells, with or without attendant thrombosis and sometimes with hemorrhage distal to the occlusion. In the past, such obstructions have been attributed to predominantly mechanical aspects of an increased blood concentration of white cells, such as an increased whole blood viscosity.[8,9] However, a reduced hematocrit keeps whole blood viscosity in the normal range in most leukemia patients[10,11] unless it is raised by ill-advised red cell transfusion[12] before the white cell count has fallen.

More recent studies emphasize reduced deformability, cytokine secretion, and altered adherence properties of blasts or other primitive cells compared with the mature cells that normally circulate.[2,13] Such factors could explain not only why leukostasis correlates more closely with the circulating blast count than with total white cell count, but also the patient-specific variability in the absolute blast count at which symptoms occur.[14] Leukostasis is seen in about 5% of patients with acute myelogenous leukemia (AML).[8] Autopsy studies have revealed microscopic correlates of leukostasis in a majority of AML patients whose white cell count exceeded 200,000/μL.[15] In most other clinically evident cases of leukostasis the blast count exceeds 100,000/μL, but the syndrome is occasionally suspected in patients with a blast count in the 50,000 to 100,000/μL range.[14] Leukostasis is uncommon in acute lymphocytic leukemia and is not expected unless the white cell count reaches the 250,000 to 300,000/μL range.[13] Higher cell concentrations, usually in the 300,000 to 500,000/μL range, are required for the more mature cells that circulate in CML to cause symptoms of leukostasis,[9] and even higher counts may be tolerated without symptoms in chronic lymphocytic leukemia.[2]

Hyperleukocytosis is also a marker for a poorer prognosis in acute and chronic leukemia, even in patients who do not present with leukostasis. Both short- and long-term survivals correlate inversely with white cell count at diagnosis, as does response to therapy expressed either as complete remission rate or duration or response.[16] Finally, hyperleukocytosis is associated with an increased risk for hyperuricemia and other manifestations of tumor lysis syndrome, which may be exacerbated by cytotoxic chemotherapy for leukemia.[17]

Despite the lack of controlled studies, it is widely accepted on the basis of accumulated clinical experience that lowering the white cell count by leukapheresis can reverse symptoms of leukostasis, even though it may not always do so. This is the basis for the ASFA/AABB ranking of hyperleukocytosis as a Category I indication for leukapheresis (Table 5).[6,7] Thus, leukapheresis should be performed emergently for leukemia patients with signs of leukostasis, especially acute leukemia patients whose blast counts exceed 100,000/µL. Wide acceptance of this principle has suggested to some that prophylactic leukapheresis might be a prudent maneuver in acute leukemia patients with white cell or blast counts of 100,000/µL or greater who do not present with symptoms of leukostasis. Although the evidence for benefit from such prophylactic leukapheresis is controversial, urgent leukapheresis may be requested routinely on this basis by individual physicians or as institutional policy, and repeated leukapheresis may be requested for acute leukemia patients whose white cell count is expected to remain high for several days before chemotherapy is instituted.[13,14] An extreme example of the latter would be a female patient who wishes to continue a pregnancy for weeks or months, in the hope of delivering a viable infant, before beginning treatment.[18]

It remains unclear whether prophylactic leukapheresis to lower the white cell count before initiation of chemotherapy can prevent or meaningfully reduce the severity of tumor lysis syndrome. A counterargument to the intuitive prediction of such benefit is that circulating leukemic cells represent only a small fraction of total tumor burden and that a meaningful reduction in the latter is unlikely to be achieved by leukapheresis. Controlled studies that address this point are lacking. Also uncertain is whether prophylactic leukapheresis could improve survival in patients with hyperleukocytosis, either by ameliorating tumor lysis syndrome or by some other mechanism.

Three observational studies of prophylactic leukapheresis have been published in the past 8 years. One group reported 48 consecutive AML patients who received leukapheresis routinely for a white cell count greater than 100,000/µL. The extent to which the white cell count was lowered by leukapheresis did not differ significantly between the 14 patients who died within 2 weeks and the remaining patients who survived longer.[19] Another nonrandomized, retrospective study of 146 patients with AML and a white cell count above 50,000/µL showed an advantage in 2-week survival for patients who underwent leukapheresis (13% vs 23%; statistically significant only in a logistic regression analysis). However, subsequent follow-up showed no advantage in 4-week, 6-week, or overall survival; long-term survival was, paradoxically, significantly less likely among patients who underwent leukapheresis.[20] A third study tabulated outcomes of 53 patients with AML and a white cell count greater than 100,000/μL who underwent daily leukapheresis (76 procedures total) as a matter of routine until the white cell count was less than 100,000/μL or performance status improved. Only two patients died in the first week. No other short-term survival data were provided; however, 47% developed coagulopathy and 85% developed tumor lysis syndrome, which was severe in 53%. Only 55% achieved a complete remission and median survival in those responders was only 8 months.[21]

Taken together, these reports do not provide strong confirmation of benefit from routine prophylactic leukapheresis in AML patients with hyperleukocytosis. They might equally well suggest that hyperleukocytosis is a marker for other risk factors, such as morphologic category, specific chromosomal abnormalities, and/or total tumor burden, that cannot be addressed simply by lowering the white cell count. Prospective randomized controlled studies are warranted.

Technique

Therapeutic leukapheresis can be performed with most centrifugal apheresis instruments. Emergent leukapheresis in patients with inadequate peripheral venous access may require equally emergent placement of a dual-lumen central venous catheter, which can be challenging in an acutely ill patient with thrombocytopenia. When deciding whether leukapheresis is appropriate for a patient who does not have the leukostasis syndrome, the clinician should balance the possible benefits of the procedure against the risks of emergent central line placement and the possible detriment that may arise from delays in implementing pharmacologic cytoreduction with hydroxyurea and in starting definitive chemotherapy.[13,14]

The efficiency of cell removal will be improved in most cases by the addition of HES or another sedimenting agent to patient blood entering the centrifuge. Also, because circulating leukemic cells may constitute a substantial fraction of blood volume, their removal, even in a leukocyte concentrate containing 500,000 to 750,000 cells per µL, may entail substantial plasma losses. The volume-expanding properties of a sedimenting agent can offset some of this loss, but additional volume replacement may be prudent when the volume of leukocyte concentrate removed approaches or exceeds one liter.[2]

The extent of prophylactic leukocyte removal that might be required to reduce the severity of tumor lysis or improve survival is, of necessity, unknown. Similarly, the extent of white cell count lowering needed to reverse or prevent leukostasis will not be known with certainty in advance for any individual case. Nevertheless, one may reasonably expect to improve the clinical situation for a patient with leukostasis if the white cell count is promptly reduced by 30% to 50%, preferably to less than 100,000/µL in AML or less than 300,000/µL in CML. As mentioned above, it is difficult to predict the extent of reduction simply on the basis of volume of blood processed.[2] It is therefore prudent to monitor STAT intraprocedural white cell counts to ensure that a targeted reduction is achieved.

Photopheresis

Extracorporeal photochemotherapy (ECP), or photopheresis, is a multistage process in which patient MNCs separated by an apheresis device are exposed to a standardized dose of ultraviolet A (UVA) radiation in the presence of a photoactive compound called 8-methoxypsoralen (8-MOP) at a concentration of 60 to 200 ng/µL. This results in crosslinking of complementary strands of nuclear DNA in the treated cells by means of diadducts between proximate thymidine residues. Some protein changes occur as well. Following a short incubation, the treated cells are reinfused to the patient. Although the apheresis and irradiation steps are conceptually independent, the modules performing them can be housed in a single instrument such as the UVAR XTS system

(Therakos, Exton, PA). 8-MOP was originally given to patients orally before apheresis but is now available in a sterile solution suitable for intravenous (IV) administration that can be added directly to the MNC concentrate just before UVA irradiation. This provides excellent control of the 8-MOP concentration during the irradiation step and lowers the dose of 8-MOP received by the patient by 100-fold, thereby reducing side effects. ECP is typically performed on 1 or 2 consecutive days at 2- to 4-week intervals in most of the applications discussed below.[22]

Cutaneous T-Cell Lymphoma

ECP was originally devised in the 1980s as a treatment for CTCL, in which malignant lymphocytes are typically found circulating in the bloodstream as well as infiltrating the skin. Certain skin manifestations of CTCL were already known to respond to removal of malignant cells by leukapheresis and also to UVA irradiation of skin after 8-MOP ingestion (psoralen-UVA treatment or PUVA). Removal, irradiation, and reinfusion of 5% to 10% of circulating MNCs on 2 consecutive days each month led to unprecedented disease regression in some patients, albeit usually after a delay of some months. The magnitude of responses cannot be explained solely by destruction of extracorporeally irradiated tumor cells, which has suggested the possibility that ECP somehow elicits, enhances, or otherwise modulates host immune responses to the tumor.[22,23] This hypothesis, in turn, has provided the basis for trials of ECP in other diseases for which immunomodulation seemed an attractive approach to therapy.

Of 282 CTCL patients reported in nine North American studies, 18% had a complete response and 38% had a partial response. Long-term follow-up of treated patients suggested a better median survival than that seen in historical controls. ECP seems most effective in patients with relatively recent onset of diffuse skin disease (erythroderma) and relatively little disease-induced immunosuppression. Results are less favorable in patients with longstanding disease, localized skin plaques, and/or involvement of lymph nodes and viscera.[23,24]

The original UVAR system was approved by the Food and Drug Administration (FDA) in 1987 for treatment of CTCL, which has been rated a Category I indication for ECP (Table 5).[6,7] Unfortunately, although its efficacy is well established, the optimal role of ECP in this most favorable indication remains uncertain because, unlike almost all strictly pharmacologic therapies for cancer, it has never been subjected to controlled trials, with uniform enrollment and response criteria, comparing it to no treatment, sham ECP, or alternative therapies.

Graft-vs-Host Disease (GVHD)

GVHD most often occurs following allogeneic stem cell transplantation. It affects predominantly the skin, the liver, and gastrointestinal tract. Acute GVHD begins before day 100 after transplant and tends to be more inflammatory, while chronic GVHD begins after day 100 and may include scleroderma-like skin thickening and other fibrotic changes. Both forms occur with regularity in allograft recipients despite prophylactic treatment with corticosteroids and other immunosuppressive drugs. The incidence of each form is about 30% following HLA-matched sibling transplants and 50% to 80% following partially mismatched related or matched unrelated transplants.[25]

Improvement in skin GVHD is sometimes seen after PUVA therapy. ECP was tried in the hope of addressing visceral involvement as well and has been reported helpful in both acute and chronic GVHD, with the best responses noted in skin manifestations.[22,26] Among 76 patients mentioned in 11 reports on acute GVHD, 83% of those with skin disease had improvement following ECP, with a complete response in 67%. Complete regression occurred in 54% of cases with gastrointestinal involvement and 38% of those with liver disease. In 20 reports on chronic GVHD, 76% of a combined 160 patients with skin disease improved after ECP, with a complete response in 35%. Improvement was reported in 48% of 84 patients with liver involvement, 39% of 31 patients with lung disease, and 63% of 59 patients with oral manifestations. Improvement is noted sooner in this context than in CTCL, with apparent responses being evident in a matter of weeks. Survival is also thought to be improved.[25] Again, however, the precise contribution of ECP to treatment of GVHD is uncertain, because patients who receive

ECP are generally receiving other therapies as well, and no prospective controlled trials have been reported. GVHD has not been rated by ASFA or AABB as an indication for ECP.

Solid Organ Transplant Rejection

Immunomodulation with ECP has also been attempted in patients who are rejecting an organ transplant. Several case studies and small series have described recipients of kidney and lung transplants, some of whom have improved when ECP was added to the anti-rejection regimen. However, the largest experience has come from heart transplantation.

The concept of rejection has a subtle additional connotation in heart transplantation that does not apply to other allografts. The latter are biopsied only when there are signs of organ dysfunction; however, the relative ease of endomyocardial biopsy (EMB) compared with renal or lung biopsy permits a transplanted heart to be biopsied routinely, often in the absence of any sign of cardiac dysfunction. It is customary for patients with normal hemodynamics who have mild histologic changes in such biopsies to be treated preemptively and aggressively for rejection. Early reports of ECP in cardiac allograft recipients described patients with severe, hemodynamically significant rejection who improved after ECP was added to other anti-rejection therapies.[22] Subsequently, a controlled trial with eight patients in each study arm found ECP to be equivalent to high-dose corticosteroids in reversing mild histologic changes on EMB.[27] However, other studies have suggested that such changes usually resolve without adjustments to anti-rejection therapy.[28] A controlled trial of prophylactic ECP in 60 patients with cardiac transplants showed a lower incidence of mild histologic changes in ECP-treated patients but no difference in the rate of severe rejection with hemodynamic compromise.[29] In the absence of controlled trials in patients with severe rejection, uncertainty about the prognostic significance of mild histologic changes contributes to uncertainty about the proper role for ECP in treatment of rejection of heart and other organ transplants. Cardiac allograft rejection has been rated as a Category III indication for ECP by ASFA and AABB (Table 5).[6,7]

Autoimmune Diseases

Immunomodulation with ECP has been tried in scleroderma, systemic lupus erythematosus, pemphigus vulgaris, rheumatoid arthritis, and psoriatic arthritis. Favorable results have been reported in case studies and small series. Further experience in scleroderma has indicated limited benefit, while definitive data from controlled studies of ECP in other autoimmune disorders are still awaited.[22]

Mechanism of Action

The mechanism of action of ECP is not known with certainty for any of the applications discussed above. There is no doubt, however, that ECP leads to apoptosis in a majority of treated lymphocytes but not in treated monocytes. UVA-induced DNA cross-linking by 8-MOP is probably an important contributor to this effect, although other mechanisms may operate as well. In CTCL, it is supposed that, as a result of apoptosis of malignant lymphocytes, antigens specific to the tumor cell clone are released or exposed in a manner that renders them more immunogenic, thereby eliciting or enhancing a host immune response to the tumor. More recent evidence suggests that contact with plastic surfaces in the apheresis device and the UVA irradiation apparatus induces monocytes in the MNC concentrate to differentiate into dendritic cells. Activated dendritic cells might then ingest tumor-specific antigens released from apoptotic cells and facilitate the antigen presentation step needed for enhanced immunity.[23,24]

A similar mechanism can be envisioned for other applications of ECP; namely, a down-regulating response to a nonmalignant but nonetheless pathogenic lymphocyte clone is enhanced through release of clone-specific antigens by apoptosis and vigorous presentation of these antigens by newly minted dendritic cells.[26,30] This mechanism should be regarded as hypothetical at present, however. Circulating clonal lymphocytes have been found in scleroderma[31] and GVHD,[26] but neither pathogenicity nor down-regulation by ECP has been demonstrated for such clones. The putative effects of ECP in GVHD have also been attributed to a more general immunomodulatory effect, evident in a shift from an inflammatory Th1 cytokine expression profile to a more inhibitory Th2 profile, and to a paradoxical decrease in dendritic cell function in this context.[26]

Hematopoietic Progenitor Cell Collection

Autologous MNCs, collected by leukapheresis and cryopreserved, have virtually replaced those derived from marrow for autologous hematopoietic rescue after myeloablative antitumor therapy for myeloma, lymphomas, leukemias, and other malignancies.[32] A similar approach is being investigated for some autoimmune diseases.[33] In the basal state, hematopoietic stem and progenitor cells (HPCs) do not circulate in quantities sufficient for this purpose; however, they can be mobilized into the bloodstream in several ways. One is to give a moderate dose of an appropriate chemotherapeutic agent ("mobilizing chemotherapy") 10 to 14 days before leukapheresis. During recovery from leukopenia, the blood concentration of CD34+ cells (a marker for HPC content) rises as much as 25-fold and remains elevated for several days. Another method is to administer hematopoietic growth factors. Both granulocyte colony-stimulating factor (filgrastim, Neupogen, Amgen, Thousand Oaks, CA) and granulocyte-macrophage colony-stimulating factor (sargramostim, Leukine, Amgen) can produce worthwhile levels of circulating CD34+ cells after four or five daily injections, and with continued daily injections this mobilization will persist for several days. In the autologous setting, growth factors can be given simultaneously in addition to mobilizing chemotherapy for theoretically maximal mobilization. Several other cytokines have also been shown to mobilize HPCs, but none is currently commercially available.[34]

Goals for autologous HPC collection at different centers range from 2 to 5 × 10^6 CD34+ cells per kg per transplant. Most patients are mobilized well enough to reach their goal after one to three daily leukapheresis procedures. A smaller proportion with marginal mobilization may require four or five daily collections. Perhaps 10% of patients, who tend to be older and/or to have had extensive prior chemotherapy, will fail to have a useful response to mobilizing stimuli. Their blood CD34+ cell levels (expressed in cells/μL) do not rise above the low single-digit range, and daily leukapheresis procedures cannot produce an adequate yield during the limited duration of the mobilization event.[34]

HPCs collected by apheresis (HPC-A) are preferred over cells derived from marrow (HPC-M) for two reasons. One is that the collection events do not require hospitalization or general anesthesia. The other is that white cell and platelet counts reach milestones of recovery about 1 week sooner after transplantation with HPC-A. The attendant reduction in early morbidity and mortality more than compensates for a somewhat higher incidence of GVHD.[32]

Candidates for HPC-A collection have distinctive requirements for vascular access. They will need a tunneled, multilumen central venous catheter to facilitate chemotherapy infusions, fluid maintenance, and transfusion support in both the pre- and posttransplantation periods. However, catheters designed solely for these purposes, albeit more comfortable, will be too small and too flexible to support the flow rates needed for leukapheresis. Fortunately, catheter manufacturers now offer tunneled dual- or triple-lumen apheresis catheters (eg, Raaf catheter) that accommodate both HPC-A collection and the full range of IV infusion therapies. Prospective autologous HPC-A transplant recipients generally should have such a catheter placed. The exception would be a patient in remission having a precautionary collection that would only be used in the event of relapse ("harvest and hold"). Such a patient should undergo leukapheresis via peripheral veins if possible.

HPC-A collections are long and extensive apheresis procedures, with 15 to 30 L of patient blood processed over 4 to 6 hours. They may cause platelet loss sufficient to warrant platelet transfusion in patients who are already thrombocytopenic. They entail prolonged infusion of citrate anticoagulant and, therefore, a large cumulative citrate dose. There have been conflicting reports regarding the frequency of adverse effects during HPC-A collection. One multicenter survey, which included both autologous and allogeneic donors but did not track either mild paresthesias or calcium replacement practices, found only a 1.33% incidence of adverse effects in 664 HPC-A collections.[35] A later, single-center study found a 54% incidence of symptoms in carefully questioned donors, in association with 20% to 35% decreases in serum ionized calcium, during 71 allogeneic HPC-A collections performed without IV calcium supplementation. Symptoms were especially prevalent in smaller female donors. The same group found a 20% incidence of symptoms among 244 donations with IV calcium supplementation, with a 10% to 15% decrease in ionized serum calcium.[36] This would suggest that IV calcium supplementation might prevent mild paresthesias during autologous HPC-A collections as well, especially in smaller females.

Autologous MNCs Manipulated Ex Vivo

Autologous MNCs collected by leukapheresis provide the starting material for a number of established and experimental cellular therapies. The remainder of this chapter briefly covers processes based on purification, expansion, immunization, and gene insertion.

Purification and Expansion

Purification of MNC subsets has been extensively explored in the setting of autologous stem cell transplantation, especially for the purpose of eliminating tumor cell contamination in autografts. In positive selection approaches, HPCs are isolated from other MNCs, including any contaminating tumor cells; immunologic techniques that target the CD34 antigen are the most prevalent and are commercially available. In addition to a lower tumor cell content, highly purified stem cells offer an attractive starting material for ex-vivo expansion techniques that might improve the outcome of transplantation in a number of ways. Negative selection techniques, in contrast, attempt to deplete tumor cells from the MNC concentrate. Positive and negative selection approaches need not be mutually exclusive.[37] Tumor cells derived from autograft contamination have been shown to be present in metastases after transplantation[38]; however, to date, no purification technique has been shown to enhance posttransplant survival in any setting.

Immunization

Several ex-vivo strategies have been proposed for inducing and/or enhancing expression of antimicrobial or antitumor activity by autologous immunocytes derived from MNC concentrates. The rationale is that enhanced antigen presentation, release from in-vivo inhibitory influences, and/or selective stimulation by supraphysiologic "cytokine cocktails" could facilitate immune responses of a type or magnitude that could not be achieved in vivo and that would produce favorable clinical effects after reinfusion of the treated cells. Such approaches have shown promise in melanoma, renal cell carcinoma, and prostate cancer.[39]

Gene Insertion

Autologous HPCs collected by leukapheresis are regarded as attractive targets for gene insertion techniques. They are easily obtained in relative abundance, and they and their progeny have the potential to survive indefinitely after genetic alteration and reinfusion. Early successes in correcting immunodeficiency resulting from adenosine deaminase deficiency were encouraging; however, gene therapy has since proven to be a very challenging endeavor.[40]

References

1. Burgstaler EA. Current apheresis instrumentation. In: McLeod BC, Price TH, Weinstein R, eds. Apheresis: Prin-

ciples and practice. 2nd ed. Bethesda, MD: AABB Press, 2003:95-130.

2. Hester J. Therapeutic cell depletion. In: McLeod BC, Price TA, Weinstein R, eds. Apheresis: Principles and practice. 2nd ed. Bethesda, MD: AABB Press, 2003:283-94.

3. Schafer AI. Thrombocytosis and essential thrombocythemia. In: Beutler E, Lichtman MA, Coller BS, et al, eds. Williams hematology. 6th ed. New York: McGraw-Hill, 2001:1541-9.

4. Greist A. The role of blood component removal in essential and reactive thrombocytosis. Ther Apher 2002;6:36-44.

5. Cortelazzo S, Finazzi G, Ruggieri M, et al. Hydroxyurea for patients with essential thrombocythemia and a high risk of thrombosis. N Engl J Med 1995;332:1132-6.

6. McLeod BC. Clinical applications of therapeutic apheresis. J Clin Apheresis 2000;15:1-5.

7. Smith JW, Weinstein R, Hillyer KL for the AABB Hemapheresis Committee. Therapeutic apheresis: A summary of current indication categories endorsed by the AABB and the American Society for Apheresis. Transfusion 2003;43:820-2.

8. Lichtman MA, Liesveld JL. Acute myelogenous leukemia. In: Beutler E, Lichtman MA, Coller BS, et al, eds. Williams hematology. 6th ed. New York: McGraw-Hill, 2001:1047-84.

9. Lichtman MA, Liesveld JL. Chronic myelogenous leukemia and related disorders. In: Beutler E, Lichtman MA, Coller BS, et al, eds. Williams hematology. 6th ed. New York: McGraw-Hill, 2001:1085-123.

10. Lichtman MA. Rheology of leukocytes, leukocyte suspensions and blood in leukemia. J Clin Invest 1973;52:350-8.

11. Steinberg MH, Charm SE. Effect of high concentration of leukocytes on whole blood viscosity. Blood 1971;38:299-301.

12. Harris AL. Leukostasis associated with blood transfusion in acute myeloid leukemia. Br Med J 1978;1:1169-71.

13. Porcu P, Cripe LD, Ng EW, et al. Hyperleukocytic leukemias: A review of pathophysiology, clinical presentation and management. Leuk Lymphoma 2000;39:1-18.

14. Porcu P, Farag S, Marcucci G, et al. Leukocytoreduction for acute leukemia. Ther Apher 2002;6:15-23.

15. McKee C, Collins R. Intravascular leukocyte thrombi and aggregates as a cause of morbidity and mortality in leukemia. Medicine 1974;53:463-78.

16. Dutcher JP, Schiffer CA, Wiernik PH. Hyperleukocytosis in adult acute non-lymphocytic leukemia: Impact on remission rate and duration and survival. J Clin Oncol 1987; 9:1364-72.

17. Davidson MB, Thakkar S, Hix JK, et al. Pathophysiology, clinical consequences and treatment of tumor lysis syndrome. Am J Med 2004;116:546-54.

18. Caplan SN, Coco FV, Berkman EM. Management of chronic myelocytic leukemia in pregnancy by cell pheresis. Transfusion 1978;18:120-4.

19. Porcu P, Danielson CF, Orazi A, et al. Therapeutic leukapheresis in hyperleucocytic leukaemias: Lack of correlation between degree of cytoreduction and early mortality rate. Br J Haematol 1997;98:433-6.

20. Giles FJ, Shen Y, Kantarjian HM, et al. Leukapheresis reduces early mortality in patients with acute myeloid leukemia with high white cell counts but does not improve long-term survival. Leuk Lymphoma 2001;42:67-73.

21. Thiébaut A, Thomas X, Belhabri A, et al. Impact of pre-induction therapy leukapheresis on treatment outcome in adult acute myelogenous leukemia presenting with hyperleukocytosis. Ann Hematol 2000;79:501-6.

22. Foss FM. Photopheresis. In: McLeod BC, Price TH, Weinstein R, eds. Apheresis: Principles and practice. 2nd ed. Bethesda, MD: AABB Press, 2003:623-42.

23. Zic JA. The treatment of cutaneous T-cell lymphoma with photopheresis. Dermatol Ther 2003;16:337-46.

24. Knobler R, Girardi M. Extracorporeal photochemoimmunotherapy in cutaneous T cell lymphoma. Ann N Y Acad Sci 2001;941:123-38.

25. Dall'Amico R, Messina C. Extracorporeal photochemo-therapy for the treatment of graft-versus-host disease. Ther Apher 2002;6:296-304.

26. Foss FM, Gorgun G, Miller KB. Extracorporeal photo-pheresis in chronic graft-versus-host disease. Bone Marrow Transplant 2002;29:719-25.

27. Costanzo-Nordin MR, Hubbell EA, O'Sullivan EJ, et al. Photopheresis versus corticosteroids in the therapy of heart transplant rejection. Preliminary clinical report. Circulation 1992;86:242-50.

28. Lloveras JJ, Escourrou G, Delisle MB, et al. Evolution of untreated mild rejection in heart transplant recipients. J Heart Lung Transplant 1992;11:751-6.

29. Barr ML, Meiser BM, Eisen HJ, et al. Photopheresis for the prevention of rejection in cardiac transplantation. Photopheresis Transplantation Study Group. N Engl J Med 1998;339:1744-51.

30. Fimiani M, Di Renzo M, Rubegni P. Mechanism of action of extracorporeal photochemotherapy in chronic graft-versus-host disease. Br J Dermatol 2004;150:1055-60.

31. French LE, Lessin SR, Kathakali A, et al. Identification of clonal T cells in the blood of patients with systemic sclerosis. Arch Dermatol 2001;137:1309-13.

32. Kessinger A. Clinical features of autologous and allogeneic peripheral blood progenitor cell transplantation. In: McLeod BC, Price TH, Weinstein R, eds. Apheresis: Principles and practice. 2nd ed. Bethesda, MD: AABB Press, 2003:493-502.

33. Burt RK, Slavin S, Burns WH, Marmont AM. Induction of tolerance in autoimmune diseases by hematopoietic stem cell transplantation: Getting closer to a cure? Int J Hematol 2002;76(Suppl 1):226-47.

34. Mechanic SA, Krause D, Proytcheva MA, Snyder EL. Mobilization and collection of peripheral blood progenitor cells. In: McLeod BC, Price TH, Weinstein R, eds. Apheresis: Principles and practice. 2nd ed. Bethesda, MD: AABB Press, 2003:503-30.

35. McLeod BC, Price TH, Owen H, et al. Frequency of immediate adverse effects associated with therapeutic apheresis. Transfusion 1999;39:282-8.

36. Bolan CD, Cecco SA, Wesley RA, et al. Controlled study of citrate effects and response to IV calcium administration during allogeneic peripheral blood progenitor cell donation. Transfusion 2002;42:935-46.

37. Meagher BC. Peripheral blood progenitor cell graft engineering. In: McLeod BC, Price TH, Weinstein R, eds. Apheresis: Principles and practice. 2nd ed. Bethesda, MD: AABB Press, 2003:545-63.

38. Brenner MK, Rill DR, Moen RC, et al. Gene marking and autologous bone marrow transplantation. Ann N Y Acad Sci 1994;716:204-14.

39. Ribas A, Butterfield LH, Glaspy JA, Economou JS. Current developments in cancer vaccines and cellular immunotherapy. J Clin Oncol 2003;21:2415-32.

40. Klein HG. Cellular gene therapy. In: McLeod BC, Price TH, Weinstein R, eds. Apheresis: Principles and practice. 2nd ed. Bethesda, MD: AABB Press, 2003:643-56.

THERAPEUTIC PLASMA EXCHANGE

Introduction

Therapeutic plasma exchange (TPE) has been successfully used to treat many hematologic, neurologic, renal, rheumatic, and metabolic disorders. In most clinical situations, it is used to remove a pathogenic or toxic macromolecule, such as an antibody, an abnormal plasma protein, or other substance. The therapeutic objective is to reduce the circulating levels of these molecules to ameliorate the disease process. TPE is also performed to replace a substance that is normally present in plasma, whose absence is deleterious to the patient. The American Society for Apheresis (ASFA)[1] and AABB[2] have grouped the indications for TPE into four categories based on the evidence supporting therapeutic efficacy: standard therapy for the disease (Category I), second-line therapy with evidence favoring efficacy (Category II), inadequate evidence for evaluation (Category III), and no demonstrated efficacy in controlled trials (Category IV). This chapter reviews many of the most frequent indications for TPE.

Hematologic Disorders and Dysproteinemias

As a group, hematologic disorders constitute one of the most common indications for TPE.[3] TPE is used to reduce levels of antibodies or immunoglobulins and to acutely replace deficient proteins involved in the pathogenesis of immunohematologic diseases. It is used as primary therapy in thrombotic thrombocytopenic purpura (TTP). In other hematologic disorders, TPE is mainly employed on an adjunctive basis, to reduce the time needed to achieve a therapeutic response or if primary pharmacologic therapy is ineffective. In light of the paucity of controlled clinical trials, guidelines published by AABB and ASFA are a valuable aid in making treatment decisions (see Table 6).

Thrombotic Microangiopathies: Thrombotic Thrombocytopenic Purpura, Adult Hemolytic Uremic Syndrome, and HELLP Syndrome

Thrombotic Thrombocytopenic Purpura

Thrombotic microangiopathies are syndromes of microangiopathic hemolytic anemia and thrombocytopenia associated with platelet aggregation in the microcirculation. In TTP, involvement of the brain and kidney produce characteristic clinical findings that include fluctuating neurologic changes and renal insufficiency. Although it is customary to consider patients who present with a predominantly neurologic picture as having TTP and those who present with renal failure as having hemolytic uremic syndrome (HUS), clinical overlap is common. For this reason, some authors prefer the combined term TTP/HUS.[4] TTP may occur on an idiopathic ("primary") basis or in association with a heterogenous group of conditions including pregnancy, autoimmune disorders, infections, and with the use of certain medications ("secondary"). Plasma exchange is the mainstay of therapy, leading to a dramatic reduction in mortality, from more than 90% to less than 20% in idiopathic TTP. Earlier recognition of cases and changes in the diagnostic threshold for treatment has led to a seven-fold increase in the number of patients treated by TPE from 1981 to 1997.[1,4]

Pathophysiology. The cardinal pathologic lesion in TTP consists of microvascular occlusion of terminal arteries and capillaries. The deposits contain platelet aggregates and von Willebrand factor (vWF) without significant amounts of fibrin or evidence of inflammation, unlike disseminated intravascular coagulation (DIC) and vasculitis, respectively. However, small amounts of fi-

Table 6. ASFA and AABB Indication Categories for Therapeutic Apheresis in Hematologic Diseases and Dysproteinemias

Disease	ASFA/AABB Category
ABO-incompatible marrow transplant	II
Aplastic anemia	III
Autoimmune hemolytic anemia	III
Coagulation factor inhibitor	II
Cryoglobulinemia	II
HELLP syndrome (postpartum)	NR
Hemolytic uremic syndrome	III
Hyperviscosity syndrome/multiple myeloma	II
Immune thrombocytopenic purpura	II*
Platelet alloimmunization	III
Posttransfusion purpura	I
Pure red cell aplasia	III
Red cell alloimmunization	III
Thrombotic thrombocytopenic purpura	I

*This disorder is ranked only in context of staphylococcal protein A immunoadsorption. NR = Disorder not ranked by either AABB or ASFA. HELLP = hemolysis, elevated liver enzymes, and low platelets. Category I = standard acceptable therapy; Category II = available evidence suggests efficacy; Category III = available evidence is inconclusive; Category IV = ineffective in controlled trials.

brin may be present when the kidney is predominantly involved, as found in HUS.[5]

Unusually large vWF multimers (ULvWF) found in the plasma of patients with TTP can directly bind to platelets via glycoprotein Ib-IX receptors, inducing platelet aggregation and the formation of microthrombi that lodge in small vessels.[5] The origin of ULvWF has recently been elucidated. Under physiologic conditions, vWF is released from endothelial cells as ULvWF. ULvWF multimers bind to the P selectin receptors on endothelial cells where they are clipped by a vWF-cleaving protease—ADAMTS13 (A Disintegrin And Metalloprotease with Thrombospondin type I motifs)—under high sheer conditions present in flowing blood. The higher-molecular-weight forms of vWF have greater adhesive properties resulting in the promotion of platelet-platelet and platelet-subendothelial interactions. Mutations in the gene for ADAMTS13 have been found to be the cause of chronic relapsing (familial) TTP. Of note, only homozygotes with a severe deficiency of protease have been reported to develop the TTP syndrome. Although most patients present during childhood, some do not develop the clinical syndrome until early adulthood. Therefore, a severe deficiency of the protease is necessary but not sufficient for the development of TTP. Other events, perhaps involving endothelial activation, may be necessary to produce the full-blown clinical disorder.[5]

In acquired or idiopathic TTP, deficiency of ADAMTS13 has been associated with IgG inhibitors in 44% to 83% of the cases.[5,6] Studies have also reported that severe deficiency of ADAMTS13 (<5%) appears to be specifically associated with idiopathic TTP,[5-7] the most homogeneous TTP subgroup. It is important to note that TTP patients with moderate deficiency (between 5% and 50% of normal), and even those with normal levels of ADAMTS13 may improve with treatment regimens that include plasma exchange.[7,8] Thus, at the present time, TTP remains a clinical diagnosis. However, the use of ADAMTS13 measurements may be helpful to predict the clinical course and to determine prognosis. Additionally, patients in whom an inhibitor is found may be considered the best candidates for the use of intensive immunosuppressive therapy.[8]

Clinical Manifestations. The full-blown "pentad" including thrombocytopenia, microangiopathic hemolytic anemia, fever, neurologic changes, and renal dysfunction, is present in only a minority of patients. A "dyad" of thrombocytopenia and microangiopathic hemolytic anemia, in the absence of another etiology, is sufficient to consider TTP as a provisional diagnosis.[4] Neurologic manifestations include headache, confusion, fluctuating sensorimotor deficits [transient ischemic attacks (TIAs)], visual defects, and seizures. The transient nature of some of the early symptoms probably reflects acute deposition and regression of microthrombi in small cerebral vessels. Coma at the time of presentation is reported to be an adverse prognostic indicator.[9] The spectrum of renal involvement ranges from proteinuria and hematuria to severe azotemia requiring dialysis. The patients who present with severe renal impairment with few neurologic or other systemic findings may be classified as having sporadic or epidemic HUS. The latter may be associated with bloody diarrhea caused by enterotoxigenic *Escherichia coli* or *Shigella* species (see section below, Adult HUS). It is important to note that TTP is a multisystem disease and other organ systems are frequently involved. Gastrointestinal ischemia (presenting with abdominal pain), acute pancreatitis, and myocardial ischemia and/or infarction have also been noted.

Laboratory studies reveal an increase in serum lactate dehydrogenase (LDH) level and the presence of schistocytes (red cell fragmentation) on a peripheral blood smear. Schistocytes reflect an active microangiopathic hemolytic process: fragmentation results from the passage of red cells through partially occluded vessels. However, early in the disease course, red cell morphology may be normal.[10] Although LDH is released from red cells as the result of hemolysis in TTP, the major portion in blood is the result of tissue ischemia secondary to microvascular occlusion.[4] Tests of coagulation generally are within normal limits. However, mild elevations of D-dimers and fibrin degradation products may be found. The following laboratory studies are recommended at the time of presentation: complete blood count and review of peripheral blood smear, reticulocyte count, prothrombin time (PT), activated partial thromboplastin time (aPTT), fibrinogen level, and D-dimer test, tests of renal and liver function, electrolytes, urinalysis, and direct antiglobulin test (DAT).

Treatment and the Role of TPE. Table 7 summarizes the results of TPE in five selected studies of patients with TTP. The majority of the patients in the studies cited had TTP as their primary diagnosis. The overall response rate was 83% with mortality of 17%. Early recurrence of disease following achievement of

Table 7. Clinical Studies: Thrombotic Thrombocytopenic Purpura

Study	Response (%)	Refractory (%)	Exacerbation (%)	Late Relapse (%)	No. of TPEs
Rose/Eldor, 1987	30/38 (79)	8/38 (21)	NA	12/30 (40)	NA
Onundarson, 1992	21/27 (78)	6/27 (22)	7/27 (22)	2/27 (7)	7-19 (mean)
CASG, Rock, 1992	40/51 (78)*	11/51 (22)*	NA	17/63 (27)[†]	16 (median)
USTTP, Banderenko/ Brecher, 1998	103/115 (90)	12/115 (10)	25/103 (24)	13/103 (13)	NA[‡]
Vesely, 2003[§]	38/48 (83)	10/48 (21)	17/38 (45)	8/38 (21)	17 (median)
Total	232/278 (83)	46/278 (17)	49/168 (29)	52/261 (20)	

*Plasma exchange arm only.
[†]Includes both arms of study, plasma exchange and plasma infusion.
[‡]Remission rate 70% by day 21; "30%... additional 1-2 weeks to respond."
[§]Idiopathic TTP-HUS only.
TPE = therapeutic plasma exchange. Exacerbation = recurrent thrombocytopenia and resumption of TPE during hospitalization (Onundarson), within 2 weeks of discontinuing TPE (USTTP), or within 1- 30 days of achieving remission (Vesely).

response (exacerbation) is fairly frequent, averaging 29%. Exacerbation was defined somewhat differently in these studies; either within a few days of stopping TPE, within 2 weeks of stopping; or within 30 days of achieving remission. If the patient remains in remission for 30 days or so after discontinuation of apheresis, recurrence is unlikely. However, approximately 20% of the patients develop a late relapse months to years after successful treatment.

Of the studies listed in Table 7, the only randomized trial was the study conducted by the Canadian Apheresis Study Group (CASG). These investigators compared plasma infusion (30 mL/kg on the first day, followed by 15 mL/kg on each subsequent day) with plasma exchange (1.5 plasma volumes per day for 3 days followed by 1.0 plasma volume per day thereafter) and demonstrated a survival advantage in the plasma exchange arm: 78% vs 63%.[11] The study established plasma exchange as the standard of care for the management of TTP. In addition to replacing missing ADAMTS13 enzyme, plasma exchange delivers a higher plasma dose (three-fold greater than plasma infusion) with greater cardiovascular tolerance and removes antibodies to ADAMTS13 that have been associated with idiopathic acquired TTP. The CASG study also demonstrated a faster clinical response by day 9 in the plasma exchange group—82% vs 49%. On average, 15.8 TPE treatments were required including five treatments tapered over a 2-week period after attainment of clinical remission.

Prompt recognition of TTP and initiation of TPE are essential because this disorder can be rapidly progressive, and delay has been shown to adversely affect outcome.[9] If a delay is unavoidable, plasma infusion (15 to 30 mL/kg daily) may be given until TPE can be performed. Guidelines for TPE generally include a 1.0 to 1.5 plasma volume exchange daily, using fresh frozen plasma (FFP) replacement until clinical symptoms resolve and there is normalization of the platelet count ($\geq 150,000/\mu L$) for at least 2 days. The LDH level should also be followed carefully because this enzyme reflects tissue ischemia. Because LDH is a nonspecific indicator, however, a slight abnormality (ie, ~ 1.5 times normal) may be acceptable at discontinuation of TPE. Once remission is obtained, some centers choose a tapering schedule in light of the 20% rate of exacerbation shortly after discontinuation of TPE. However, a recent retrospective study found no significant difference in the rate of relapse when comparing taper and no-taper apheresis schedules.[12]

Unless serious bleeding occurs, platelet transfusions are contraindicated because they may exacerbate platelet microvascular deposition that might lead to rapid clinical deterioration or a neurologic event, such as a TIA. Fortunately, serious hemorrhage is unusual in TTP.

As mentioned above, FFP is the standard replacement solution for patients with TTP. Plasma, Cryoprecipitate Reduced (cryo-poor plasma or cryosupernatant) contains ADAMTS13 and can be used as an alternative. This product has the theoretical advantage of containing reduced levels of vWF, which is involved in platelet adhesive interactions. Although several small, uncontrolled reports suggest a benefit, a recent small, randomized clinical trial found no difference in outcome in comparison to FFP.[13]

Two broad groups of agents have been used as adjuvant pharmacologic therapy for TTP: 1) antiplatelet agents and 2) immunosuppressive medications (a recently completed evidence-based review is recommended for more complete information).[10] Antiplatelet agents have not proved to be particularly effective in the treatment of TTP, and the risk of hemorrhage may be increased, particularly in patients with severe thrombocytopenia. The thienopyridine derivatives (ticlopidine, clopidogrel) have been associated with drug-induced TTP; ticlopidine has been shown to induce autoantibodies to ADAMTS13. These agents should not be used. A growing body of evidence points to autoimmunity as the etiologic basis for idiopathic TTP, renewing interest in the use of immunosuppressive agents. The role of glucocorticoids remains uncertain with comparable mortality rates reported in the literature.[4] If not used initially, they are frequently introduced later if the response to TPE is unsatisfactory. Vincristine may be useful as a second-line agent. A regimen of 1 mg given intravenously, repeated every 3 to 4 days with a total of four doses, has been recommended in refractory TTP.[10] Cyclophosphamide and cyclosporine have also been tried in refractory cases. More recently, the anti-CD20 monoclonal antibody rituximab has been introduced. Reports using the drug at conventional doses of 375 mg/m^2 on a weekly basis for 4 to 8 weeks have shown responses in the majority of treated patients.[14] An unresolved issue concerns the dosing schedule of the drug, which has a half-life of 21 days. It is unclear whether removal of the drug by plasma exchange affects its overall efficacy. Therefore, it is prudent to administer rituximab immediately after TPE if it is used. In the case series reported, time until remission averaged between 2 and 5 weeks and appeared to be sustained. Splenectomy has also been utilized, primarily in patients with frequent relapses of TTP. This approach has been shown to reduce the attack rate from an average of 2.3 ± 2.0 events/year to 0.1 ± 0.1 event/year in a retrospective case series.[15]

Technical Issues. FFP is the replacement fluid of choice because of replenishment of missing ADAMTS13 and/or other enzymes, which may be important in processing vWF. Plasma, Cryoprecipitate Reduced is a suitable alternative. Shortages of one or the other may require use of both on an ongoing basis. If both are in short supply and the patient has an uncommon blood type—for example, AB or B—it may be necessary to perform the first part of the exchange with albumin and reserve plasma for the second half of the exchange. This approach has been used routinely by one institution with good results overall.[12] Platelet transfusions are relatively contraindicated except for serious hemorrhage. Red cell transfusions can be given if required.

Some secondary causes of TTP do not respond as rapidly, have a lower response rate, and have poorer survival than idiopathic TTP.[7] Patients with clinical features of TTP in the setting of cancer, cancer-chemotherapy, and stem cell transplantation respond poorly to therapy and the role of TPE is not established. Treatment of TTP is classified by both ASFA and AABB as a Category I indication for TPE.[1,2]

Adult Hemolytic Uremic Syndrome

Adult HUS presents as acute renal failure in association with microangiopathic hemolytic anemia and thrombocytopenia. The disease may be associated with enterocolitis, neurologic sequelae, liver dysfunction, pancreatitis, and cardiac ischemia, making it difficult to distinguish from TTP.[16,17] Idiopathic HUS, both in adults and children, may be further classified into typical (or epidemic) and atypical. Epidemic HUS is associated with verotoxin-producing bacteria including *E. coli* O:157H:7, or other verotoxin-producing organisms such as *Shigella* species. Epidemic HUS (also called diarrhea positive, or "D+") is the most common cause of HUS in children; conversely, it occurs in the minority of adult cases.

Thrombocytopenia tends to be not as severe in HUS as in TTP. For example, in one series the mean platelet count was 36,000/µL in patients classified as having HUS compared with 18,000/µL in those having TTP.[7] In another, platelet counts averaged 95,000/µL in HUS and 35,000/µL in TTP.[18] ADAMTS13 levels are generally normal or slightly decreased with only rare HUS patients having severe deficiency.[8] Moreover, most reports have shown an absence of inhibitors in patients with HUS. Further support for a diagnosis of HUS vs TTP may be found in renal biopsy specimens. Arterial and capillary thrombosis is prominent in TTP, and thrombi stain strongly for platelets and vWF. In comparison, the typical histologic changes in HUS consist of glomerular and arteriolar fibrin thrombi and subendothelial widening of the glomerular capillaries on electron microscopy.[10]

Treatment of epidemic HUS generally involves supportive measures including control of high blood pressure and volume status, and dialysis as needed. Antibiotics may exacerbate or prolong the disease and should be avoided. Epidemic HUS in adults occurs in the elderly with serious neurologic complications and has a poor prognosis. Although small case series have reported efficacy,[19] there is no clear-cut role for TPE in the management of epidemic or nonepidemic HUS in adults.[10] However, a therapeutic trial may be considered if there is any doubt in distinguishing between HUS and TTP. HUS is classified as a Category III indication for TPE by both ASFA and AABB.[1,2]

HELLP (Hemolysis, Elevated Liver Enzymes, and Low Platelets) Syndrome

The HELLP syndrome presents during pregnancy or in the peripartum period as a manifestation of preeclampsia. HELLP must be distinguished from TTP or HUS occurring during pregnancy, which accounts for approximately 13% of the female patients in case series of TTP.[20] In a review of TTP in pregnancy, 30% of cases presented during the third trimester, when preeclampsia, eclampsia, and HELLP syndrome occur, and 47% presented after delivery. Fever is usually not present in preeclampsia and HELLP syndrome, whereas it may be present in TTP or HUS. Although ADAMTS13 levels are reduced in the third trimester of pregnancy, HELLP syndrome is not associated with severe deficiency as seen in TTP.[20]

HELLP occurs in up to 10% of women with severe preeclampsia.[17] Thrombocytopenia and abnormal liver function studies (ie, increased transaminase levels) can also present without the significant hypertension and proteinuria that are typical of preeclampsia. HELLP manifestations can also appear as much as 6 days after delivery.[10] Typical presenting symptoms include nausea, abdominal pain, and edema. Maternal mortality in HELLP syndrome is less than 1%; however, there is an associated 10% to 20% infant mortality rate caused by placental ischemia that results in abruption or prematurity.[10] There is no clear benefit to the use of corticosteroids; expedited delivery is the treatment of choice for severe preeclampsia and for HELLP syndrome, and usually leads to rapid recovery of platelets, often within 24 to 48 hours.

Limited retrospective studies suggest that TPE is effective if performed in patients with persistent evidence of disease 72 hours or more following delivery or when there is serious organ compromise, including liver, kidney, lungs, or central nervous system (CNS).[21] Patients in the favorable group generally have a platelet level near or above 50,000/μL and recovered platelets to above 100,000/μL by the sixth postpartum day in comparison with patients with platelet nadirs below 50,000/μL, who required up to 11 days to achieve the 100,000/μL level. Overall mean recovery time in the plasma exchange group was 6.5 days, similar to those with the less severe HELLP. Thrombocytopenia in the favorable group responded rapidly with one or two TPE treatments. In comparison, the response was variable in nine patients complicated by single or multiple organ failure. The patients with a septic process were at high risk and failed to respond to TPE; there were two deaths in this group.[22] TPE does not appear to be effective in patients with preeclampsia or eclampsia syndrome without HELLP.[23,24]

The role of TPE in HELLP syndrome is unclear. It has not been classified by AABB or ASFA. More severe thrombocytopenias tend to respond quickly to plasma exchange, but it is uncertain if this prevents more severe complications. Management of acute respiratory distress syndrome, sepsis, and the complications of DIC carry preeminent importance in the care of these complex patients.

Autoimmune Hemolytic Anemia

Warm and cold autoimmune hemolytic anemias are so named because of the thermal characteristics of the antibodies involved. Warm (IgG) autoantibodies bind to red cells maximally at 37 C, whereas 4 C is generally the temperature of maximal reactivity for IgM antibodies. The differences in antibody characteristics result in distinct clinical syndromes. Rare IgG cold-agglutinins have also been reported.

Warm-Antibody Hemolytic Anemia (WAHA)

WAHA occurs in both a primary (idiopathic) and secondary form [eg, systemic lupus erythematosus (SLE), lymphoproliferative disorders] and represents 70% of all autoimmune hemolytic anemias. Females predominate in a proportion of 3:1. The onset of hemolysis may be gradual or abrupt. Typical symptoms include weakness, fatigue, dyspnea on exertion, jaundice, and a low-grade fever. The DAT is positive for IgG alone or IgG plus complement. Reticuloendothelial cells bearing Fc receptors, located primarily in the spleen, clear IgG-coated red cells. Several factors influence the severity of hemolysis, including antibody concentration, the avidity of antibody binding to red cell antigens (usually directed to components of the Rh complex), the ability to fix early components of the complement cascade, as well as the functional capacity of the reticuloendothelial system itself.

Initial treatment consists of high doses of corticosteroids (1-2 mg/kg prednisone) in an attempt to block reticuloendothelial clearance of the coated red cells. Other immune-modulating agents reported to be useful include intravenous immunoglobulin (IVIG), cytotoxic drugs (such as cytoxan), rituximab, and splenectomy. Judicious transfusion management is essential.

TPE has been used in fulminant or drug-refractory patients with limited success and has been classified as a Category III indication by ASFA and AABB.[1,2] Intensive plasma exchange may be necessary for sufficient antibody removal because of the large volume of distribution of IgG autoantibody. In case reports and case series, stabilization of active hemolysis has been reported.[17,25,26] Silberstein reported two patients who received three plasma exchanges resulting in a decreased red cell transfusion requirement; however, with use of autologous labeled red cells, the red cell half-life following the TPEs was unchanged. Two studies reported beneficial responses employing TPE followed by either IVIG or cytoxan in highly refractory patients.[17] TPE is generally reserved for fulminant cases of WAHA, especially after failure of immunosuppressive therapy. A reasonable approach would be to use 1.0 to 1.5 plasma volumes on a daily to every-other-day basis, for a total of four to six treatments.

Cold-Antibody Hemolytic Anemia (CAHA)

CAHA may also occur as an idiopathic disorder or in association with lymphoproliferative disorders or certain viral or mycoplasma infections. Red cell sludging may induce acral cyanosis in the colder portions of the body, including the ears, nose, and tips of the digits. IgM autoantibodies in this disorder typically have anti-I specificity and bind to red cells at lower body temperatures where they avidly fix complement. Upon recirculation to warmer core temperatures, the IgM dissociates, leaving complement-only coated red cells that are cleared predominantly in the liver. The DAT is positive for complement. The thermal amplitude and titer of cold agglutinins largely determine their clinical behavior: antibodies reactive at temperatures closer to normal body temperatures are more likely to cause hemolysis.

Corticosteroids are generally ineffective except in low-titer cases. Immunosuppressive agents used include chlorambucil, cytoxan, azathioprine, and, more recently, rituximab.[17,27] A warm ambient temperature should be maintained as well as utilization of a blood warmer for all transfusions.

The predominant intravascular distribution of IgM allows for efficient removal by TPE. Substantial reduction in cold antibody titers and improved labeled red cell survival have been demonstrated in response to TPE, in conjunction with clinical improvement.[28] The risk of ex-vivo agglutination and worsening anemia may be minimized by use of a blood warmer in the TPE circuit. A single case-report describes the use of synchronized therapy with cytoxan after successive TPE.[29] Overall, TPE may be useful in severe cases of CAHA to temporarily reduce the titer and activity of the cold antibodies. The temperature of the extracorporeal circuit should be maintained as close to body temperature as possible to prevent iatrogenic anemia from clumping and loss of red cells in the cell separator. CAHA is classified as a Category III indication for TPE by ASFA and AABB.[1,2]

Immune Thrombocytopenic Purpura

Immune mechanisms similar to those involved in WAHA may also cause thrombocytopenia. In adults, immune thrombocytopenic purpura (ITP) follows a chronic relapsing and remitting course that is typical of autoimmune disorders. Approximately three times more females than males are affected with a peak incidence in the third to fourth decade. Onset may be sudden and severe, but more commonly it develops insidiously. Patients may complain of easy bruising, gingival bleeding, and excessive menstrual bleeding over a period of several months.

The platelet antibodies involved in the pathogenesis of ITP are directed against platelet surface glycoprotein antigens, primarily glycoproteins IIb/IIIa and Ib/IX. Diagnostic platelet antibody testing has not been shown to be clinically useful. The diagnosis is suggested by the finding of isolated thrombocytopenia, large or "young" platelets on peripheral blood smear, normal or increased numbers of megakaryocytes on marrow examination (if performed), and the absence of alternative causes for destructive thrombocytopenia such as sepsis, DIC, or TTP/HUS.

Therapy is based on the assessment of bleeding and the severity of the platelet count. Corticosteroids (1-2 mg/kg/day of prednisone or equivalent) are employed initially, followed by tapering to reduce the incidence of long-term side effects. Individuals who are steroid resistant or require excessive doses may respond to additional therapies including IVIG, IV Rh Immune Globulin in D-positive patients, splenectomy, danazol, vincristine, or other immunosuppressive agents such as rituximab.

Evidence suggesting a role for TPE in the management of ITP is scant, consisting of a few case reports[26] and a single small clinical trial that suggested a lower relapse rate in patients who received both TPE and steroids.[30] A beneficial effect was also reported in two noncontrolled studies that coupled the use of TPE and IVIG.[31,32] Bussell, employing TPE on 3 consecutive days followed by IVIG 1 g/kg/day × 2 days, observed a response in four of eight patients refractory to IVIG and prednisone. The mean peak platelet increment was 132,000/μL (range 74,000 to 225,000/μL). The response was temporary, however, with platelets dropping to baseline within 2 weeks. Responses were seen only in patients who had previously responded to IVIG.

TPE treatment of ITP has not been classified by AABB or ASFA; however, the use of SPA immunoadsorption (discussed in Chapter 6) has been classified as a Category II indication.[1,2] A consensus committee formed by the American Society of Hematology has concluded that, in ITP, TPE should be considered only in severe cases refractory to steroids and splenectomy.[33]

Posttransfusion Purpura

Posttransfusion purpura (PTP) is a rare syndrome characterized by the sudden onset of severe thrombocytopenia with platelets less than 10,000 to 20,000/μL occurring 5 to 14 days after blood transfusion. Most cases are associated with red cell transfusions. The thrombocytopenia is self-limited, eventually resolving within 2 to 6 weeks. Women are predominantly affected, likely the result of sensitization to platelet-specific antigens during pregnancy. Sensitization usually involves the HPA-1a antigen; other platelet-specific antigens have also been reported. The development of a brisk alloantibody response is associated with profound thrombocytopenia, despite the absence of the inciting antigen on the patient's own platelets. Several explanations have been offered in an attempt to explain this finding, including antigen adsorption from the transfused HPA-"incompatible" blood and the detection of circulating IgG autoantibodies.[17]

Transfusions of HPA-incompatible platelets are generally ineffective. HPA-compatible platelets may be effective,[34] but they are seldom available on an emergent basis.

The immunopathogenesis of this condition has spurred various therapeutic approaches. There are no controlled clinical studies; therefore, it is difficult to evaluate their true efficacy. Corticosteroids appear to shorten the duration of thrombocytopenia.[35] IVIG has also been reported to be efficacious, sometimes within hours of administration.[17] Responses to IVIG have been seen after failure of steroids and TPE.[36]

Before the advent of IVIG, both exchange transfusion and TPE appeared to be effective based on historical results.[34,37] In some cases, thrombocytopenia recurred and improved after resumption of TPE. Given the rapidity and durability of responses using IVIG, this agent has become the mainstay of therapy for PTP. IVIG also avoids certain risks associated with the TPE procedure, especially the need for central venous catheterization in some patients, and dilutional coagulopathy. If TPE is utilized in the small proportion of patients unresponsive to steroids and/or IVIG, close attention should be paid to coagulation screening tests; FFP replacement may be needed to avoid dilutional coagulopathy because of the need for daily intensive apheresis. PTP has been classified as a Category I indication by both ASFA and AABB.[1,2]

Coagulation Factor Inhibitors

Inhibitors to specific coagulation factors may develop on an autoimmune or alloimmune basis. Alloantibodies against Factor VIII complicate the management of 15% to 20% of patients with severe hemophilia A. Spontaneous Factor VIII autoantibodies may also develop in patients with autoimmune disorders such as SLE, in the elderly, or as a complication of pregnancy. Serious, potentially fatal bleeding episodes may ensue from this form of "acquired hemophilia." Immunosuppressive agents consisting of corticosteroids, cytoxan, and rituximab have been used to eradicate Factor VIII autoantibodies Coagulation products that promote hemostasis are also frequently needed, depending upon the nature and degree of hemorrhage.

Hemostatic coagulation products are indicated for treatment of bleeding episodes or in preparation for surgical procedures. Establishing a normal level of Factor VIII is considered the optimal approach, if possible. However, this is practical only in the small percentage of cases with low-titer inhibitors (eg, <5 Bethesda units/mL). High doses of human Factor VIII may be needed to overcome the inhibitor. In the majority of patients, products containing activated coagulation factors (FEIBA, Baxter, Vienna, Austria; NovoSeven, NovoNordisk, Princeton, NJ) are used to "bypass" the inhibitor. These approaches may fail, however, leading to efforts to reduce the inhibitor titer utilizing TPE followed by Factor VIII infusion.

Experience using TPE in factor inhibitor patients consists of uncontrolled small case series and case reports. Slocombe described successful management of a Factor VIII deficient hemophilia patient who developed postoperative bleeding caused by a new onset Factor VIII inhibitor.[38] Fourteen TPEs consisting of 4 liters each were performed daily, resulting in 90% reduction in inhibitor and apparent cessation of bleeding in response to Factor VIII infusion. Transient (less than 24 hours) increases in Factor VIII levels were documented. Another hemophilia A patient with Factor VIII antibodies underwent successful drainage of a psoas muscle abscess despite Factor VIII inhibitor titers as high as 203 Bethesda units (15 units using porcine Factor VIII).[39] TPE on two separate occasions resulted in lowering the inhibitor titer to 4 Bethesda units (porcine) and therapeutic levels of Factor VIII were achieved using bolus and continuous infusion of porcine Factor VIII.

Case reports also describe the use of TPE in patients with acquired Factor VIII inhibitors in conjunction with immunosuppressive therapy (steroids, cytoxan, and Factor VIII concentrate), with successful resolution of hemorrhage.[40] TPE has also been reported to be useful in other types of coagulation factor inhibitors including those to Factors V and X, thrombin, and vWF.[26,41] Immunoadsorption columns have also been used (see Chapter 6).

Multiple courses of TPE may be necessary to achieve a reduction in the titer of the IgG inhibitors in these patients. FFP replacement is indicated to avoid dilutional coagulopathy. Considering the largely anecdotal evidence of benefit and the availability of increasingly effective and safe coagulation products, the risks associated with placement of a central catheter are difficult to justify in these patients. Coagulation inhibitors are listed as a Category II indication by ASFA and AABB.[1,2]

Dysproteinemias

This category refers to a group of disorders with excessive or aberrant immunoglobulin production. The abnormal proteins may either be monoclonal (eg, produced by a malignant clone of plasma cells as in Waldenström's macroglobulinemia) or polyclonal (as seen in cryoglobulinemia and SLE). Several disorders that are relevant to TPE practice are discussed here.

Hyperviscosity Syndrome

An elevated viscosity occurs in up to 50% to 70% of patients with Waldenström's macroglobulinemia, a B-cell lymphoproliferative disorder characterized by the hyperproduction of monoclonal IgM molecules.[17] Increased serum viscosity is related both to individual aggregating characteristics of the molecule as well as the quantitative level. In its full expression as the hyperviscosity syndrome, elevated serum viscosity leads to hypervolemia with a range of neurologic manifestations—headache, dizziness, vertigo, nystagmus—eventually leading to somnolence, stupor, and coma. Retinal hemorrhages with exudates are frequent, at times resulting in visual impairment. There also is an associated coagulopathy related to impaired platelet function and fibrin polymerization.[42] Hyperviscosity syndrome has also been observed in up to 5% of patients with multiple myeloma, (predominantly IgA and less commonly IgG) and even more rarely in patients with benign polyclonal B-cell proliferations, eg, SLE and rheumatoid arthritis.

Relative serum viscosity is quantified by measuring the time it takes for serum to travel through a glass tube in comparison to water. Normal values range from 1.5 to 1.8 Ostwald units. Symptomatic hyperviscosity syndrome is usually not seen until relative serum viscosity exceeds 4 Ostwald units. Most patients with values between 5 and 8 Ostwald units are symptomatic, and nearly all patients with levels beyond 8 Ostwald units have symptoms. The relationship between protein concentration and viscosity is not linear; rather, viscosity increases exponentially as serum protein concentration increases. Therefore, a relatively small reduction in protein concentration from TPE may result in a dramatic improvement in symptoms. This is especially noteworthy because the expanded plasma volume results in underestimation of plasma volume by standard calculations.[17]

Few TPE applications show as rapid a symptomatic response as hyperviscosity syndrome. The patient's sensorium may improve dramatically during the procedure as a result of increased capillary blood flow and cerebral perfusion. It has been estimated that reducing the total IgM level by 15% to 20% with removal of 1000 mL of plasma reduces the relative viscosity by more than 50%.[42] Definitive chemotherapy treatment is indicated, however, because these effects on mental status, bleeding symptoms, visual impairment, and hypervolemia are temporary. Patients who are no longer responding to drug therapy may be effectively managed by chronic regular TPE.[43]

In Waldenström's macroglobulinemia, a single 1.0 to 1.5 plasma volume TPE procedure involving 50% to 80% albumin/20% to 50% normal saline replacement is generally sufficient to lower serum viscosity to the normal range. This is due to the predominantly intravascular distribution of IgM. Hyperviscosity syndrome due to IgG or IgA multiple myeloma or polyclonal proteins may require more treatment. The course should be tailored to symptomatic response and serum protein measurements. AABB and ASFA classify hyperviscosity syndrome as a Category II indication.[1,2]

Multiple myeloma affects individuals (predominantly males) older than 40 years. Manifestations include anemia and other cytopenias, bone pain, and fractures related to osteoporosis and plasmacytomas. Hypercalcemia is also frequently seen. Renal failure complicates the clinical course in over half of the patients with multiple myeloma and is a serious prognostic indicator. In most cases, acute reversible causes of renal failure are sought, including dehydration, hypercalcemia, IV contrast nephropathy, and infection. In addition to these causes, renal failure may result from renal tubular injury secondary to the light chain deposition or amyloidosis. The reversibility of this form of renal injury has been the subject of several case series and two controlled clinical trials.

Recognition that light chains are toxic to renal tubules has spurred various efforts at removal. Hemodialysis is relatively inefficient. Peritoneal dialysis is somewhat better; however, it is less effective than TPE.[44,45] Uncontrolled studies suggest that aggressive management of the underlying condition, including chemotherapy, dialysis, and TPE, may improve prognosis.[46,47] Misiani et al reported recovery of renal function in eight of 10 patients with acute renal failure, including normalization of serum creatinine in five patients and improvement in 11 of 13 patients with chronic renal failure. TPE, 35 mL/kg, was performed on days 1 to 5 of each cycle of chemotherapy (cytoxan plus prednisone). Although median survival of the entire group of patients was short (9 months), there was no difference in survival between those with acute renal failure and chronic renal failure and those with complete vs incomplete recovery of renal function.

In a randomized controlled clinical trial, 29 patients with acute renal failure (24 receiving dialysis) were randomly assigned to receive TPE, corticosteroids, cytotoxic treatment, and hemodialysis if needed, or to a control arm receiving corticosteroids, cytotoxic drugs, and peritoneal dialysis.[48] Renal function improved (creatinine <2.5 mg/dL) in 13 of 15 patients in the TPE arm of the study vs only two of 14 patients in the non-TPE arm. These findings were paralleled by reduction in light chain excretion in the TPE arm only. Survival was also significantly improved in the TPE group: 66% vs 28%. This study has been criticized because the two groups were treated differently, not just in TPE but also in the use of hemodialysis vs peritoneal dialysis.[49] In another randomized study, 21 patients (12 requiring hemodialysis) with progressive renal failure received either 1) melphalan and prednisone plus forced diuresis or 2) melphalan and prednisone plus TPE (given 3 times per week for 1 to 4 weeks). The average time was about 6 weeks from recognition of renal dysfunction to protocol treatment. Although there was no overall difference in the two groups in renal function recovery or survival, three of seven TPE patients who required dialysis were able to discontinue it vs none of five control patients. The light chain levels were reduced rapidly in the TPE group.

In patients with multiple myeloma, early recognition of renal dysfunction and determination of medically reversible causes is paramount. A renal biopsy may assist in determining whether irreversible renal lesions exist, such as severe cast formation or amyloidosis, with little possibility of reversal by TPE. Patients with less severe cast formation or tubular interstitial changes may be the best candidates for reversal of nephropathy by TPE. Renal failure due to multiple myeloma is classified as a Category II indication by ASFA and AABB.[1,2]

Cryoglobulinemia

Cryoglobulins are proteins that precipitate with cold exposure and dissolve with rewarming. Three types are recognized. Type 1 cryoglobulins are monoclonal proteins, usually found in association with multiple myeloma. Type 2 "mixed" cryoglobulins are monoclonal proteins (usually IgM) that have bound polyclonal IgG. Type 3 cryoglobulins consist of polyclonal immunoglobulin/antigen complexes. Types 2 and 3 are associated with systemic vasculitis, and clinical findings include leukocytoclastic angiitis (manifested as "palpable" purpura), polyarthralgias, glomerulonephritis, neuropathy, skin ulceration, and cold intolerance. Type 2 cryoglobulins are often found in the context of chronic hepatitis C infection.

Treatment is directed at alleviating the vasculitic manifestations. Drugs used include corticosteroids (provided viral hepatitis is excluded) and immunosuppressives. TPE has been employed to lower the concentration of cryoglobulins. A direct relationship exists between the concentration of cryoglobulins and their precipitation characteristics, with higher levels precipitating at higher temperatures.[50] Therefore, lowering the levels may reduce symptomatic manifestations involving the skin and joints and may also protect the kidneys.[51] Chronic regular or intermittent TPE may provide long-term control of the disease, particularly if drug therapy is toxic or ineffective. Cryoglobulinemia is classified as a Category II indication by ASFA and AABB.[1,2]

Neurologic Diseases

Several neurologic diseases affecting both the peripheral and the central nervous systems have been associated with the presence of autoantibodies. Although the pathogenic nature of these autoantibodies may not have been definitively established in each case, TPE has been used with clinical success in the treatment of several of these neurologic diseases.[1,2] (See Table 8.)

Guillain-Barré Syndrome

Guillain-Barré syndrome is a progressive neurologic disease affecting the peripheral nervous system. It is acute in onset and often follows an infectious illness. Patients frequently present with progressive lower-extremity weakness, loss of tendon reflexes, and paresthesias, progressing to involvement of the upper extremities and face. Ultimately, patients may require ventilatory support. Some patients have dysautonomic symptoms as well, including blood pressure lability. Symptoms may worsen for up to 4 weeks, but generally improve after that time. This limited time course may help distinguish Guillain-Barré syndrome from the more pro-

Table 8. ASFA and AABB Indication Categories for Therapeutic Apheresis in Neurologic Disorders

Disease	Procedure	ASFA/AABB Category
Guillain-Barré syndrome	Plasma exchange	I
Chronic inflammatory demyelinating polyneuropathy	Plasma exchange	I
Polyneuropathy with IgG/IgA monoclonal protein	Plasma exchange	I
Polyneuropathy with IgM monoclonal protein	Plasma exchange	II
Myasthenia gravis	Plasma exchange	I
Stiff-person syndrome	Plasma exchange	III
Lambert-Eaton myasthenic syndrome	Plasma exchange	II
Paraneoplastic neurologic syndromes	Plasma exchange	III
Polymyositis or dermatomyositis	Plasma exchange Leukapheresis	III IV
Multiple sclerosis	Plasma exchange	III
Idiopathic inflammatory demyelinating disease	Plasma exchange	II
Refsum's disease	Plasma exchange	III
Rasmussen's encephalitis	Plasma exchange	III
Sydenham's chorea	Plasma exchange	II
PANDAS (pediatric autoimmune neuropsychiatric disorders associated with streptococcal infections)	Plasma exchange	II

Category I = standard acceptable therapy; Category II = available evidence suggests efficacy; Category III = available evidence is inconclusive; Category IV = ineffective in controlled trials.

tracted timeframe of chronic inflammatory demyelinating polyneuropathy (CIDP).

The diagnosis of Guillain-Barré syndrome relies heavily on clinical findings; examination of the cerebrospinal fluid typically reveals few mononuclear cells with increased protein. Electrophysiologic studies may reveal slowed nerve conduction velocities, consistent with the loss of myelin. Several antibodies directed against gangliosides from Schwann cells and/or axons have been associated with Guillain-Barré syndrome.[52] Patients with ophthalmoplegia have been found to have antibody directed against ganglioside GQ1b, an antigen found in ocular nerves.

Guillain-Barré syndrome is a self-limited disease; however, patients often require intensive supportive care, including ventilatory support, followed by prolonged rehabilitation. Corticosteroids alone are not helpful in the treatment of Guillain-Barré syndrome. Several randomized, controlled trials have shown that TPE is effective treatment for Guillain-Barré syndrome, significantly shortening recovery time, decreasing ventilatory support needs, and decreasing disability in treated patients as compared with controls.[53]

The typical TPE treatment protocol for Guillain-Barré syndrome consists of five or six procedures over 10 to 14 days, exchanging 1.0 to 1.5 plasma volumes with each procedure and replacing with 5% albumin and saline. Patients should be reassessed at the completion of an initial course of therapy; additional procedures may be indicated in the setting of severe disease. Patients generally tolerate TPE well, although those patients with disease affecting their autonomic system may experience hypotension and blood pressure lability during TPE. Guillain-Barré syndrome is considered a Category I indication for TPE by both ASFA and AABB.[1,2]

Studies have shown a role for IVIG in the treatment of Guillain-Barré syndrome. Two randomized trials have compared the therapeutic option of IVIG vs TPE. The largest trial treated 150 patients and found that patients receiving IVIG had more rapid clinical improvement than the patients receiving TPE.[54] A smaller randomized trial by Bril et al[55] showed equivalency between the two treatment protocols as assessed by improvement in disability grade at 1 month. An international, multicenter randomized trial compared IVIG vs TPE vs a combined regimen of TPE followed by IVIG.[56] With over 120 patients in each treatment group, the authors found similar efficacy between the IVIG and TPE treatment arms. Combined therapy offered no significant advantage. Consequently, many neurologists prefer to treat patients with IVIG, because it is often a logistically less complicated approach.

Chronic Inflammatory Demyelinating Polyneuropathy

Patients with CIDP have a progressive clinical course with worsening symmetric proximal and distal weakness. The progressive clinical symptoms last for longer than 8 weeks, a distinction that separates CIDP from Guillain-Barré syndrome.[57] CIDP may be seen in the setting of other underlying diseases, including hepatitis, inflammatory bowel disease, Hodgkin's disease, connective tissue diseases, and human immunodeficiency virus (HIV) infection. CIDP may also be seen in association with a monoclonal gammopathy; this is discussed in more detail below.

The diagnosis of CIDP is largely clinical, but cerebrospinal fluid may reveal elevated protein. Evidence of demyelination, with slow conduction and conduction blocks, is seen on electrodiagnostic studies. Most nerve biopsies show histologic evidence of demyelination with an associated mononuclear inflammatory infiltrate.[58]

CIDP is presumed to be antibody mediated, because of its many similarities to Guillain-Barré syndrome and its association with monoclonal gammopathies. Although several autoantibodies have been identified in patients with CIDP, including antibodies directed against gangliosides and components of myelin, their pathogenicity has not been definitively established.[59]

Many patients respond to corticosteroid therapy. Immunosuppressive drugs, such as azathioprine, cyclophosphamide, and cyclosporine, are used in patients who do not respond to steroid treatment. IVIG has also been used with success in CIDP. Controlled trials have shown no significant difference between the clinical effects of IVIG vs TPE vs steroids.[60]

Two randomized, sham-controlled trials have demonstrated a role for TPE in the treatment of CIDP.[61,62] Both trials showed significant clinical improvement in the treated patients as compared to sham-treated controls. A frequently used plasmapheresis regimen consists of six procedures over 10 to 14 days, which may be followed by two procedures per week for 4 weeks. With each procedure, a single plasma volume is replaced with 5% albumin and saline. Many advocate the use of TPE for patients with severe disease. Both AABB and ASFA consider CIDP to be a Category I indication for TPE.[1,2]

Peripheral Neuropathy with Monoclonal Gammopathy

Monoclonal gammopathies occur when a B-lymphocyte clone is capable of producing monoclonal proteins, typically in the setting of a B-cell malignancy such as multiple myeloma or Waldenström's macroglobulinemia. When a monoclonal gammopathy is identified without the diagnostic features of myeloma or macroglobulinemia, it is considered a monoclonal gammopathy of undetermined significance (MGUS) because some of these patients may ultimately develop disease. Peripheral neuropathy has been seen in association with monoclonal proteins. The POEMS syndrome is a specific syndrome including both neuropathy and monoclonal proteins, in addition to other features (Polyneuropathy, Organomegaly, Endocrinopathy, Monoclonal protein, Skin changes).[63]

The peripheral neuropathy that is found in association with a monoclonal protein bears many similarities to CIDP; however, a few differences exist. Patients with a monoclonal protein often present with sensory symptoms, as well as motor deficits. Pathologic examination of nerve biopsies may reveal demyelination, axonal degeneration, and nerve fiber loss.[64] Autoantibodies directed against various peripheral nerve antigens have been identified in these patients.

Although patients with underlying B-cell malignancies should be treated for their malignancy, the neuropathy may not respond in parallel to the disease response. Similar to CIDP, patients with MGUS and a neuropathy are often treated with immunosuppressives. IVIG has also been used with success.[65] A sham-controlled trial demonstrated efficacy of TPE in treating patients with neuropathy in the setting of MGUS.[66] They found greater improvement in the patients with IgG or IgA monoclonal proteins as compared with the patients with IgM monoclonal proteins.

The TPE treatment protocol for these patients includes five or six procedures over 10 to 14 days, with each procedure removing a single plasma volume and replacing with 5% albumin and saline. Both AABB and ASFA consider neuropathy with IgG or IgA monoclonal protein as a Category I indication for TPE, whereas neuropathy with an IgM monoclonal protein is rated as a Category II indication.[1,2]

Myasthenia Gravis

Fatigue and weakness that worsen with activity are the clinical hallmarks of myasthenia gravis. Patients may present with ptosis and diplopia; however, many patients present with generalized weakness.[67] In the most severe instances, patients develop bulbar symptoms with difficulty swallowing, leading to the risk of aspiration. Diaphragmatic weakness can lead to respiratory compromise requiring ventilatory support.

The neurologic symptoms seen in myasthenia gravis are caused by the presence of IgG antibodies directed against the alpha subunit of the acetylcholine receptor (AChR). These antibodies can be detected in 75% to 95% of patients with myasthenia gravis.[68] The antibodies increase the turnover of the receptor, damage the junctional folds of the motor endplate, and limit the efficacy of neurotransmitter by competitive inhibition. All of these mechanisms can result in the weakness seen in myasthenia gravis. Less commonly, patients may be found to have antibodies to MuSK, a tyrosine kinase receptor that is restricted to the neuromuscular junction.[68]

The medical treatment of myasthenia gravis consists of two distinct types of therapy. Drugs that inhibit cholinesterase enzymes, such as pyridostigmine (mestinon) and neostigmine, delay the degradation of acetylcholine at the motor endplate and thereby improve strength. Immunosuppressive drugs can be helpful by reducing autoantibody production and/or by decreasing the inflammatory damage to the motor endplates.[69]

81

Many patients with myasthenia gravis will be found to have a malignant thymoma, and surgical resection can lead to neurologic improvement. In patients without thymoma, thymectomy can prove helpful, but this is controversial because of the lack of controlled studies.[69]

Several uncontrolled trials have shown that TPE is effective in the treatment of myasthenia gravis.[70,71] TPE reduces the level of antibody against AChR, which correlates with clinical improvement. TPE is recommended for the treatment of patients with myasthenia gravis in several circumstances: severe disease, disease unresponsive to medical treatment, and in preparation for surgery, including thymectomy. A frequently used treatment schedule consists of five or six treatments. In more severe cases, the initial treatments might be on consecutive days, followed by procedures every other day. With each procedure, a single plasma volume is removed and replaced with 5% albumin and saline. On occasion, patients may require longer-term maintenance TPE with ultimate tapering of procedures, as clinically tolerated. Maintenance TPE may begin at weekly intervals, which are gradually extended to 2-week intervals and ultimately progress to 4-week intervals. Myasthenia gravis is considered a Category I indication for plasmapheresis by both ASFA and AABB.[1,2]

Studies evaluating the relative efficacy of IVIG and TPE for the treatment of myasthenia have had mixed results. One retrospective trial showed that TPE led to more rapid improvement than 2.0 g/kg IVIG.[72] A randomized trial showed equivalent results for TPE and 1.2 g/kg IVIG.[73] Because neither therapy has been shown to be superior, both TPE and IVIG are used for the treatment of myasthenia. Often, IVIG is considered preferable for logistical reasons.

Lambert-Eaton Myasthenic Syndrome

Patients with Lambert-Eaton myasthenic syndrome (LEMS) present with fatigue, proximal extremity weakness, and signs of dysautonomia. These patients do not have the symptoms of ptosis, diplopia, and dysarthria that are seen in myasthenia gravis In approximately half of cases, LEMS is a paraneoplastic syndrome, often seen in association with small cell carcinoma of the lung.

The clinical symptoms seen in patients with LEMS are felt to be caused by impaired signal transduction at the neuromuscular junction. Patients with LEMS have been found to have autoantibodies directed against P/Q- and N-type voltage-gated calcium channels. These calcium channels are critical for both neuromuscular transmission and autonomic function. It is felt that the IgG autoantibodies are capable of binding the calcium channels, leading to cross-linking of channels, with disruption and ultimate reduction in number of channels.[67,74]

Cholinesterase inhibitors, which are used for the treatment of myasthenia gravis, are less effective in the treatment of LEMS. Drugs that are helpful in the treatment of LEMS include 3,4-diaminopyridine and immunosuppressives such as prednisone and azathioprine. In cases associated with a malignancy, treating the underlying tumor may be helpful. IVIG has shown efficacy when the LEMS is not associated with lung cancer. TPE has been shown to be effective in treating some patients with LEMS,[74] especially when used in conjunction with immuno-suppression. Patients who initially respond to TPE may subsequently worsen and require additional TPE treatment. Both AABB and ASFA consider LEMS a Category II indication for TPE.[1,2]

Multiple Sclerosis and Transverse Myelitis

Multiple sclerosis (MS) is a disease of the CNS in which patients experience episodes (or attacks) of neurologic dysfunction due to focal areas of demyelination. These "plaques" of demyelination can be detected by magnetic resonance imaging. In the relapsing-remitting variant of MS, patients experience intermittent attacks with intervening periods of improvement. In chronic progressive MS, patients progressively worsen over time. The waxing and waning nature of the disease makes it a particularly difficult disease to study, because spontaneous improvement can be easily confused with therapeutic effect. Although the pathogenesis of the disease is not fully understood, it is felt to be autoimmune in nature. It was previously considered a disease of the cellular immune system because of the presence of T cells in the "plaques." Recent evidence has implicated a pathogenic role for the humoral immune system in MS.[75,76] Transverse myelitis is a neurologic disease with sensory, motor, or autonomic dysfunction attributable to inflammation of the spinal cord in the absence of compression, tumor, or vascular compromise.[77]

Medical therapy for MS includes corticosteroids, adrenocorticotropic hormone, and various immunosuppressive agents. Although steroids are a mainstay of therapy for acute attacks, aimed at decreasing inflammation and edema associated with "plaques," it is unclear whether steroid therapy changes the course of the disease. Adrenocorticotropic hormone is also used to treat acute attacks. Interferon beta has been used with success to treat relapsing-remitting MS. Glatiramer acetate, which consists of amino acids contained in myelin basic protein, is used to reduce relapse rates in relapsing-remitting MS. Other immunosuppressive agents, such as cyclosporine, cyclophosphamide, and azathioprine, can also be used.[78] Steroid therapy is the treatment of choice for transverse myelitis.

In sham-controlled trials, TPE has not shown efficacy for the treatment of chronic progressive MS.[79,80] Recently, a sham-controlled crossover trial evaluated TPE in treating patients with acute severe idiopathic inflammatory demyelinating disease (IIDD), which includes both MS and transverse myelitis.[81] In these severe cases, which were refractory to steroid therapy, TPE was found to be effective therapy as compared with a control. Based on this study, patients are treated with 10 TPE procedures every other day; each procedure replaces one plasma volume with 5% albumin and saline. Although additional supportive studies would be helpful, both AABB and ASFA consider acute severe IIDD, or acute fulminant CNS demyelination, to be a Category II indication for TPE.[1,2] Relapsing-remitting MS and progressive MS are Category III indications for TPE.

Stiff-Person Syndrome

Once known as stiff-man syndrome, stiff-person syndrome is a disease characterized by progressive rigidity and/or spasms involving the trunk and proximal limbs. Patients have an antibody directed against glutamic acid decarboxylase, an enzyme required for the synthesis of gamma-amino butyric acid (GABA), a neurotransmitter for inhibitory synapses in the CNS.[82]

Medical treatment for stiff-person syndrome consists of diazepam, prednisone, drugs that increase CNS GABA levels (eg, baclofen), and IVIG.[82,83] Although no controlled trials have been performed, case reports have described successful treatment with TPE. Consequently, this is a Category III indication for TPE.[1,2]

Paraneoplastic Syndromes

Several paraneoplastic syndromes occur in which neurologic symptoms are seen in association with tumors. Sometimes, the neurologic symptoms are evident before the malignancy has been identified.[84]

In paraneoplastic cerebellar degeneration, patients develop pure cerebellar symptoms including ataxia, nystagmus, and dysarthria. This entity has been seen in association with breast and ovarian carcinomas; patients may have antibodies directed against Purkinje cell antigens.[85]

Patients with paraneoplastic encephalomyelitis present with neurologic symptoms related to a particular region of the CNS. This is seen in association with small cell carcinoma of the lung. Patients may have an antibody, anti-Hu, which has specificity for a protein associated with nuclei of both neurons and small cell cancer cells.[85]

Paraneoplastic syndromes may improve following treatment of the underlying tumor; however, this is an inconsistent result. Immunosuppressive drugs are often given, but their efficacy is inconsistent.[86] There are only case reports in the literature showing a benefit from TPE therapy.[87] Consequently, these paraneoplastic syndromes are considered Category III indications for TPE.[1,2]

Renal Diseases

Only select renal diseases respond to plasmapheresis therapy; consequently, TPE should be used only in specific clinical settings (see Table 9).[1,2] Rapidly progressive glomerulonephritis (RPGN) comprises several immune-mediated diseases of the kidney, including Goodpasture's syndrome, pauci-immune glomerulonephritis, and immune complex glomerulonephritis. These diseases are classified as RPGN because they share clinical and pathologic features. All of these diseases clinically progress at a rapid rate and, if untreated, result in end-stage renal disease. The pathologic hallmark is the finding of crescent formation on routine histology. However, the optimal treatment of these diseases differs, and TPE is not helpful in the treatment of all types of RPGN.

Goodpasture's Syndrome

Goodpasture's syndrome or antiglomerular basement membrane disease is caused by antibody directed against Type IV collagen that is present both in the glomerular basement membrane and the pulmonary alveolar basement membrane. Consequently, patients may present with signs of hematuria, proteinuria, and progressive renal failure, or they may present with pulmonary symptoms such as dyspnea and hemoptysis, or they may have a combination of renal and pulmonary signs and symptoms. Chest radiography may reveal infiltrates related to pulmonary hemorrhage. Many patients report a history of a preceding respiratory tract infection. The disease is usually self-limited, but if rapid treatment is not initiated, end-stage renal disease may result, requiring dialysis and ultimate transplantation. Additionally, the pulmonary hemorrhage may be life-threatening.

Diagnosis should include the finding of glomerular basement membrane antibodies. Routine staining of renal biopsy specimens reveals crescent formation, while immunofluoresence staining reveals linear deposition of IgG and C3. It is felt that the glomerular basement membrane antibodies are capable of activating complement, leading both to leakage of fibrin into Bowman's space with formation of crescents and to disruption of alveolar vessels, resulting in pulmonary hemorrhage.[88]

Immunosuppressive and anti-inflammatory drugs are generally given in an effort to decrease antibody production and decrease the inflammatory response. Plasmapheresis is used to reduce the pathologic antibody. A randomized study evaluated the

Table 9. ASFA and AABB Indication Categories for Plasma Exchange in Selected Renal, Rheumatic, Metabolic, and Miscellaneous Disorders

Disease	ASFA/AABB Category
Renal disorders	
Glomerular basement membrane antibody disease	I
Other rapidly progressive glomerulonephritis	II
Hemolytic uremic syndrome	III
Recurrent focal and segmental glomerulosclerosis	III
Lupus nephritis	IV
Rheumatic disorders	
Systemic vasculitis	III
Scleroderma/progressive systemic sclerosis	III
Systemic lupus erythematosus	NR
Antiphospholipid antibody syndrome	NR
Rheumatoid arthritis	IV
Metabolic disorders	
Acute hepatic failure	III
Overdose/poisoning	III
Solid organ transplantation	
Presensitization to donor organ	III
Transplantation across ABO barrier	III
Heart transplant rejection	III
Renal transplant rejection	IV

Category I = standard acceptable therapy; Category II = available evidence suggests efficacy; Category III = available evidence is inconclusive; Category IV = ineffective in controlled trials; NR = not ranked.

role of adding TPE to immmunosuppression in these patients. Patients receiving TPE had more rapid decreases in glomerular basement membrane antibodies and lower creatinine levels.[89] However, patients who present with dialysis dependence are unlikely to benefit from TPE.[90]

The recommended treatment of Goodpasture's syndrome includes cyclophosphamide, steroids, and TPE. The TPE regimen typically consists of daily procedures for 7 to 14 days or until the antibody is no longer detectable. Replacement with 5% albumin is acceptable, unless daily procedures lead to depletion of coagulation factors or during active pulmonary hemorrhage, during which time FFP should be given. Goodpasture's syndrome is rated a Category I indication for TPE by both AABB and ASFA.[1,2]

Pauci-Immune Rapidly Progressive Glomerulonephritis

Pauci-immune RPGN is usually associated with the finding of perinuclear neutrophil cytoplasmic antibodies. In addition to renal disease, patients may also have a systemic vasculitis, such as Wegener's granulomatosis or microscopic polyarteritis nodosa.

Kidney biopsies will show a crescentic glomerulonephritis. Immunofluorescence staining reveals only scant or absent staining for IgG and C3. This disease is felt to result from cell-mediated inflammation. The inflammatory process results in destruction of the glomerular capillary wall, leading to crescent formation.

The treatment of pauci-immune RPGN should focus on immunosuppressives, anti-inflammatory drugs, and cytotoxic agents. Case reports in the literature suggest a role for TPE in the treatment of this disease; however, a randomized trial was not convincing.[91,92]

Many advocate the use of TPE as adjunctive therapy during the initial presentation. Initially, daily procedures can be performed, followed by an every-other-day schedule, replacing with 5% albumin and saline. RPGN that is negative for antiglomerular basement membrane antibodies is rated as a Category II indication for TPE by both AABB and ASFA.[1,2]

Focal and Segmental Glomerulosclerosis

Focal and segmental glomerulosclerosis (FSGS) generally presents with proteinuria that progresses to nephrotic syndrome and, ultimately, to renal failure requiring dialysis and kidney transplantation. This disease can present in a primary form, or it can be secondary to various conditions such as HIV infection and heroin abuse. Several specific genetic mutations have been identified in patients with primary FSGS. FSGS has a recurrence rate in transplanted organs of approximately 20% to 40%.[93] A circulating factor has been identified in patients with this disease, suggesting a therapeutic role for TPE.[93,94]

Although generally unsuccessful, the treatment of primary and recurrent FSGS usually includes immunosuppressive agents, such as steroids, cyclosporine, azathioprine, cyclophosphamide, and mycophenolate mofetil. Angiotensin-converting enzyme inhibitors and angiotensin II antagonists have been associated with improvement in proteinuria.[93] Although there are no controlled studies evaluating the role of TPE for these patients, many case reports suggest a beneficial role for TPE. Consequently, a course of TPE in conjunction with immunosuppressive agents and an angiotensin II antagonist is often instituted soon after the diagnosis has been determined.[95] Procedures can be started on a daily schedule, followed by treatments every other day. The replacement fluid is typically 5% albumin, unless depletion of coagulation factors indicates a need for plasma replacement. AABB and ASFA consider recurrent FSGS a Category III indication for TPE.[1,2]

Solid Organ Transplantation

The use of TPE in the setting of solid organ transplantation is an area of growing interest. Despite an increasing number of patients in need, solid organ transplantation is limited by the number of available organs. In an effort to expand the pool of available organs, many groups are developing immunosuppressive and immunomodulatory protocols to facilitate incompatible organ transplantation; these protocols often include TPE.

Renal Transplantation

Routine renal transplantation requires both HLA and ABO compatibility. Consequently, patients who are HLA alloimmunized as a result of previous transplantation, transfusion, or pregnancy are less than optimal candidates for future transplantation, and it is more difficult to find a compatible donor for them.

Even patients who receive an organ from a compatible donor may ultimately develop antibody-mediated rejection on the basis of HLA antibodies. These antibodies and the resulting rejection may present any time from a week after transplantation to many years later. The rejection episode can be diagnosed by the presence of specific HLA antibodies directed against the donor and by characteristic histologic findings on kidney biopsy. Previously known as "vascular rejection," the histology of antibody-mediated rejection has recently been refined to include both features seen on routine staining and immunofluoresence staining for C4d.[96]

Four randomized, controlled trials reported between 1981 and 1990 showed no benefit for TPE in treating acute vascular rejection.[97-100] In these trials, patients were also treated with immunosuppression, including steroids, either alone or with subcutaneous heparin or cyclophosphamide. Consequently, this is considered a Category IV indication for TPE by both AABB and ASFA.[1,2]

More recently, protocols have been developed to treat antibody-mediated rejection and salvage these transplants using TPE in conjunction with more intensive immunosuppresion, including tacrolimus, mycophenolate mofetil, IVIG, and rituximab. Only case reports are available to document success in treating humoral rejection in kidney transplantation.[101] These newer studies are limited to patients with circulating donor-specific antibody and biopsies showing evidence of antibody-mediated rejection, including immunofluorescence staining for C4d.

Similar treatment protocols have been developed to enable transplantation in patients with pre-existing HLA antibodies.

When preformed antibodies are present at the time of transplant, there is a high risk of hyperacute rejection. The goals of these protocols are to remove antibody and prevent hyperacute rejection. There are numerous case reports of success, but no randomized, controlled studies. One protocol uses a series of TPE procedures followed by cytomegalovirus hyperimmune globulin both preoperatively and postoperatively in conjunction with an intensive immunosuppressive regimen.[101] The transplant procedure is performed only if a negative crossmatch is achieved. Both AABB and ASFA consider HLA sensitization before renal transplantation a Category III indication for TPE.[1,2]

ABO-incompatible kidney transplants have been performed in Japan for more than 10 years. Because of severe limitations in the availability of cadaveric organs in Japan, transplant centers there have developed protocols using immunosuppression and membrane differential filtration plasmapheresis (see Chapter 6) to facilitate ABO-incompatible kidney transplantation. Over 400 ABO-incompatible transplants have been performed in 55 transplant centers.[102] They report success, with patient and graft survival comparable to the concurrent ABO-compatible transplants. Transplant centers in the United States have begun performing ABO-incompatible transplants as well, with similar reports of success.[103,104]

Cardiac Transplantation

Cardiac transplantation requires ABO donor-recipient compatibility. There is also a growing appreciation for the role of HLA antibodies in cardiac transplantation. Consequently, there are increasing similarities between cardiac and renal transplant issues, relating to antibody-mediated rejection and removal of presensitizing HLA antibodies before transplantation.

There remains controversy surrounding the histologic diagnosis of antibody-mediated rejection in cardiac transplant biopsies. Patients can be tested for the presence of HLA antibodies and it may be possible to determine if the patient's HLA antibody is specific for the donor. When patients have signs of cardiac dysfunction and histologic evidence of humoral rejection with or without the finding of HLA antibody, many centers recommend adding TPE to the immunosuppressive regimen. No case-controlled studies have been performed, and only a few case reports describe success in the literature. AABB and ASFA consider this a Category III indication for TPE.[1,2]

When patients are known to have HLA antibodies before the transplant procedure, some centers have tried to remove the antibody. Logistically, the process is more complicated, because all donors are cadaveric and there is limited time between notification of an available organ and the time at which the organ must be transplanted. One report describes successful thoracic organ transplantation in four patients with HLA antibodies following a single TPE procedure and high-dose IVIG administration immediately before transplantation.[105]

ABO-incompatible heart transplants have been successful in infants and small children up to 14 months of age. The protocol includes immunosuppression and intraoperative use of donor-compatible plasma products, with a plasma exchange performed during cardiopulmonary bypass. It is felt that the extremely young age of the patients may allow for the induction of tolerance of the incompatible graft.[106]

Liver Transplantation

Liver transplants are routinely ABO compatible. However, ABO-incompatible liver transplants are more successful than are kidney or heart grafts. Both pre- and postoperative TPE procedures have been used with reported success in ABO-incompatible liver transplantation,[107-109] but no randomized, controlled studies have been performed.

Primary allograft nonfunction or primary dysfunction is diagnosed when failure of graft function occurs shortly after liver transplantation. This complication is associated with increased morbidity and mortality. Conventional treatment for primary allograft nonfunction is retransplantation. One case study found improved graft and patient survival with TPE treatment, obviating the need for retransplantation in several cases.[110] Another report did not show improved graft survival with TPE.[111] No randomized, controlled studies have been performed. This indication has not been categorized by AABB or ASFA.[1,2]

Rheumatic Diseases

Systemic Lupus Erythematosus and Lupus Nephritis

SLE is an autoimmune disorder in which autoantibodies and circulating immune complexes lead to complement activation and tissue destruction. The disease may involve the entire body; no organ system is spared. As is true for many autoimmune diseases, women are affected more often than men.

The diagnosis of SLE is considered when high levels of antinuclear antibodies (ANA) are found. Antibodies to double-stranded DNA (anti-dsDNA) and Sm antigen are often present as well. High levels of ANA and anti-dsDNA with complement depletion are felt to be indicative of active disease. The cause of this abnormal autoantibody production is unclear; however, it is these autoantibodies and associated circulating immune complexes that result in the organ dysfunction characteristic of SLE.[112]

Lupus nephritis is a relatively common complication of SLE Patients have deposition of immunoglobulin within their glomeruli and immunofluorescence staining of kidney biopsies reveals granular immunoglobulin and C3 deposition. This process leads to proteinuria and ultimate renal failure.

SLE is treated with immunosuppressive agents, including steroids, azathioprine, cyclophosphamide, and mycophenolate mofetil. Patients with end-stage renal disease from lupus nephritis require dialysis and should be considered for transplantation.

Although one would expect TPE to be very useful in the treatment of SLE and its complications, the results of trials have not been supportive. A randomized, sham-controlled trial of patients with mild disease showed that, although six TPE procedures over 2 weeks did reduce immunoglobulin and circulating immune complexes, there was no clinical benefit from TPE.[113] An uncontrolled trial suggests that TPE may be helpful for patients with severe disease when used in conjunction with cyclosporine.[114]

The Lupus Nephritis Collaborative Study Group conducted a controlled clinical trial involving 86 patients who were randomly assigned to receive cyclophosphamide and prednisone with or without TPE. The patients receiving TPE had decreased anti-dsDNA and circulating immune complexes. However, there was no improvement in clinical parameters with the addition of TPE.[115] Consequently, lupus nephritis is considered a Category IV indication for TPE.[1,2]

Antiphospholipid Antibody Syndrome

Patients with antiphospholipid antibody syndrome (APAS) may present with recurrent arterial or venous thrombotic events, recurrent pregnancy loss, and thrombocytopenia in the presence of antiphospholipid antibodies, such as IgG or IgM anticardiolipin antibodies. These patients frequently test positive for the lupus anticoagulant. Most patients with SLE will have antiphospholipid antibodies; however, they do not all have APAS. An entity known as catastrophic APAS is particularly aggressive with a mortality rate of approximately 50%. Patients die of multiorgan thrombosis and infarction.[116]

Patients with APAS should be anticoagulated indefinitely with warfarin. A history of arterial thromboses may indicate a need for aspirin therapy. For patients with high-titer antiphospholipid antibody who may be at increased risk for catastrophic APAS, immunosuppressive therapy such as steroids, cyclophosphamide, azathioprine, and mycophenolate mofetil should be considered. TPE should be considered in the setting of catastrophic APAS, especially when anticoagulation appears to be ineffective or is precluded by a hemorrhagic complication.[117,118] AABB and ASFA have not ranked APAS or catastrophic APAS as an indication for TPE.

Vasculitis

Systemic vasculitis includes numerous diseases in which an inflammatory process involves the vessels and ultimately leads to vascular compromise. Patients may present with fever, arthralgias, and myalgias. Many of the systemic vasculitides are associated with antineutrophil cytoplasmic antibodies (ANCA), which may have a predominance of either cytoplasmic (c-ANCA) or perinuclear (p-ANCA) distribution. Specific patterns of ANCA are more commonly associated with different diseases. For example, c-ANCA is more prevalent in Wegener's granulomatosis,[119] and p-ANCA is more commonly associated with polyarteritis nodosa, Churg-Strauss syndrome, crescentic glomerulonephritis, and Goodpasture's syndrome.

The pathophysiology of these diseases is felt to be linked to the deposition of immune complexes in the vessel walls, leading to complement activation and destruction. Therapy is aimed at decreasing the levels of ANCA and the resulting immune complexes. Immunosuppression with steroids in combination with cytotoxic drugs, such as cyclophosphamide, is the treatment of choice.

It would seem that TPE could be effective in removing ANCA and immune complexes. However, only a few controlled trials have been reported. The European Vasculitis Study Group has reported encouraging preliminary data from their randomized controlled trial of patients with ANCA positivity and RPGN. Patients treated with TPE and steroids have less dialysis dependence than patients treated with steroids alone. A study of Churg-Strauss syndrome and polyarteritis nodosa unrelated to hepatitis B infection evaluated the potential therapeutic role of TPE when added to steroid therapy; the authors found no additional benefit of TPE. In a subsequent study, the same group found that TPE did not improve the prognosis of patients with severe disease, but it did help control the disease. In hepatitis B-related polyarteritis nodosa, TPE has been shown to be effective therapy.[120]

Both AABB and ASFA consider severe systemic vasculitis to be a Category III indication for TPE.[1,2] Many centers use TPE in these patients as adjunctive therapy in the most severe cases, especially when patients are not responsive to immunosuppressive agents such as steroids and cyclophosphamide.[120] In these situations, initial therapy may include daily TPE procedures, progressing to every other day once the clinical situation has stabilized. Replacement fluid should be 5% albumin unless coagulation factor depletion or pulmonary hemorrhage would dictate the need for plasma replacement.

Metabolic Diseases

Acute Hepatic Failure

The prognosis of patients with acute hepatic failure who progress to stage 3-4 encephalopathy is poor, with historical survival rates ranging from 10% to 40%. Liver transplantation is associated with improved survival in the 60% to 80% range; however, many patients die while waiting for a donor organ to become available.[121] TPE is used in hepatic failure to correct or partially correct the coagulopathy resulting from liver dysfunction. TPE can restore the levels of deficient coagulation factors while avoiding the circulatory overload that may result from infusion of large volumes of plasma. It has also been used to allow time for hepatocyte regeneration in cases of reversible hepatic injury and to maintain the clinical status of patients waiting for liver transplant. TPE has been advocated to remove or reduce the levels of accumulated endogenous toxins believed to be associated with encephalopathy, cerebral edema, and progressive multisystem organ failure. However, it is inefficient at removal of many of the implicated toxins because of their relatively small size and large volume of distribution.[122] The most common causes of acute liver failure are acetaminophen toxicity, types A and B hepatitis, and alcohol. Other possible etiologies include fulminant Wilson's disease, reactions to drugs or toxins, and acute fatty liver of pregnancy.

Methodologic issues hamper assessment of the value of TPE in clinical studies. There have been no controlled trials assessing the role of TPE in acute hepatic failure. Uncontrolled clinical studies using "standard" TPE in disparate patient groups have reported mixed results. A 30% to 40% reduction in the levels of biochemical markers (bilirubin, ammonia) after apheresis was typically seen. No survivors were noted in nine patients with acute viral hepatitis using manual TPE.[123] In another study of nine patients, seven (77%) had improvement in coma grade and five (55%) survived.[124] However, four of the five survivors had acetaminophen-induced acute hepatic failure, which has a better prognosis. A third study reported recovery in three of four patients (viral and drug-induced hepatitis) using an aggressive (10-liter) processing regimen.[125] More recently, clinical and physiologic responses have been noted utilizing intensive "large-volume" membrane plasmapheresis (10-16 liters). Investigators reported survival in five of 11 (46%) patients in one study and 11 of 18 (61%) in another utilizing TPE followed by liver transplantation.[126,127] Improvement in encephalopathy was observed, along with a temporary increase in cerebral blood flow, but there were no changes in intracranial pressure. The lack of an effect of TPE on intracranial hypertension is notable, given the association of this complication with cerebral edema and mortality in acute liver failure.

A recent study examining the role of TPE in children with acute hepatic failure consisted of 49 patients who underwent 243 TPE procedures for various indications including acute hepatic failure, candidate for liver transplant, and coagulopathy.[128] TPE was performed daily using an average of 2.2 plasma volumes with FFP as the replacement fluid (cryoprecipitate was used in 26%). The authors observed transient neurologic improvement (mainly after initial TPE), minor changes in bilirubin, and serum ammonia. The primary benefit was an improvement in coagulopathy; no bleeding complications were observed, despite return of the PT or international normalized rate to the previous baseline by the next day. In patients with fulminant hepatic failure associated with Wilson's disease, the massive release of copper ions from necrotic liver is toxic to red cell metabolic pathways, resulting in acute hemolysis and renal impairment. TPE, using 1.0 or 2.0 exchanges, has been shown to reduce elevated serum copper levels to normal and to ameliorate the hemolytic anemia.[129]

The side effects of TPE may be quite significant in patients with acute hepatic failure who are critically ill, have low systemic vascular resistance, and are often hypotensive. Decreased metabolism of citrate may lead to potentially serious hypocalcemia (and hypomagnesemia)[130] with the possibility of tetany, seizures, cardiac irritability, depressed myocardial function, and hypotension. Close monitoring of ionized calcium levels and intravenous calcium supplementation are generally employed. In the large-volume membrane TPE procedures, heparinization is necessary to reduce the infused citrate load, potentially worsening the bleeding risk of the existing coagulopathy. FFP is necessary for coagulation factor replacement. Metabolism of the infused citrate leads to a metabolic alkalosis, which increases the equilibrium conversion of ammonium to ammonia ($NH_4^+ > NH_3$) and potential exacerbation of encephalopathy. The potential for toxicity of the apheresis procedure needs to be carefully considered in critically ill patients with acute hepatic failure.

TPE for acute hepatic failure is classified by AABB and ASFA as a Category III indication.[1,2] Its primary role is to manage severe coagulopathy, which is a frequent and challenging complication in these patients.

Drug Overdose and Poisoning

Drug overdose and poisoning represent an increasing health-care problem in the United States. Of 2.3 million poisonings in 1997, 21% required medical treatment, and 12% required intensive care unit admissions.[131] The general principles of care involve medical stabilization and toxin removal by various methods, including gastrointestinal decontamination (eg, activated charcoal), increased elimination (eg, forced diuresis), or removal from the bloodstream by various extracorporeal techniques. There is increasing availability of specific antidotes for certain toxins, eg, n-acetylcysteine for acetaminophen overdose.

Extracorporeal techniques are rarely used in the management of acute poisoning and intoxications. Protein-bound drugs/toxins with a limited volume of distribution may be more efficiently removed by TPE than other techniques, such as hemodialysis or hemofiltration. Hemodialysis is more effective for small-molecular-weight drugs with large volumes of distribution. Hemofiltration can remove drugs bound to small-molecular-weight proteins (generally less than 30,000 Daltons).

The true efficacy of TPE, or any extracorporeal method, is difficult to evaluate in light of the concomitant use of multiple potentially effective therapies and the lack of controlled trials. A number of case reports or small case series describe successful application of TPE and drug/toxin removal (Table 10). The literature also reports apparent success with agents that are not highly protein bound and have a large volume of distribution.[133] Included in this category are digitoxin, paraquat, amanita phalloides toxin, and L-thyroxine. More recent reports have

Table 10. Medications and Toxic Substances for Which Successful Use of TPE Has Been Described

Medication	P_b (%)	V_d (L/kg)	Metabolism	Excretion
Digitoxin	30	6-7	Stomach	Urine
Cisplatin	90	0.3	Liver	Urine
Vincristine	75	7.2	Liver	Feces
Verapamil*	90	4.5-7	Liver	Urine
Thyroxine*	99†	ND	Liver	Feces
Antithymocyte globulin	NA	0.12	Liver/Spleen	NA
Phenprocoumon (warfarin derivative)	99	0.14-0.17	Liver	Urine
Phenytoin*	90-95	0.6-0.7	Liver	Bile/Urine
Paraquat	0	1.2-1.6	Liver	Urine
Methylparathion	>90	10	Liver	Urine/Feces
Sodium chlorate	NA	ND	Kidney	Urine
Amanita toxin	Low	ND	NA	NA
Ethylene glycol	?	0.83	Liver	Urine

*Reports describing failure of plasma exchange were also published.
†P also reported as 25-30% in Winters.[132]
P_b = protein binding; V_d = volume of distribution; NA = not applicable; ND = not determined.
Modified from Szczepiorkowski.[133]

questioned the value of TPE in some of these cases. For example, Piqueras et al found that forced diuresis was able to remove many times more amanita phalloides toxin than TPE.[134] Other studies have reported that the use of thioctic acid, an antidote of amanita phalloides toxin, resulted in more than 80% survival, equivalent to studies in which TPE was used.[135] A recent report also describes the lack of efficacy of TPE in two patients with thyrotoxicosis.[132] Advances in medical management of this disorder and the extensive tissue distribution of L-thyroxine have led to the recommendation that TPE should be considered only in life-threatening overdoses.

Table 10 also lists drugs for which TPE treatment was reported to be ineffective. Additional drugs included in this category are barbiturates, aluminum, tricyclic antidepressants, benzodiazapines, quinine, and phenytoin.[132] TPE has also been shown to have a negligible effect upon reduction in the therapeutic levels of digoxin, digitoxin, prednisone, prednisolone, propranolol, and tobramycin. The availability of specific reversal agents for some of these drugs also has lessened the role of TPE in the management of drug toxicity.[132,136]

The role of TPE in the management of poisoning and drug overdose remains undefined, and both AABB and ASFA designate this as a Category III indication.[1,2] Toxic levels of highly protein-bound drugs and failure of medical therapy are the primary considerations in respect to a therapeutic trial of TPE. If TPE is used, an exchange consisting of at least 1.0 to 1.5 plasma volumes would be appropriate. Replacement fluid should consist of 5% albumin to ensure adequate drug/toxin removal from tissues by reequilibration. Clinical response and drug/toxin levels should be carefully monitored.

Storage Diseases

Refsum's Disease

Phytanic acid storage disease or Refsum's disease is an autosomal recessive condition resulting from the inability to break down phytanic acid—a dietary lipid. Accumulation in the body leads to the clinical disorder known as heredopathia atactica polyneuritiformis, which is characterized by multiple neurologic manifestations including retinitis pigmentosa, peripheral neuropathy, cerebellar ataxia, sensorineural deafness, and anosmia.[137] Additional findings include ichthyosis, skeletal problems, and cardiac arrhythmias. Elevation in phytanic acid occurs in relation to concurrent illnesses or weight loss, probably due to mobilization from adipose tissue.

Dietary restriction of animal sources of phytanic acid is the cornerstone of therapy for Refsum's disease. A number of case reports and/or case series have found beneficial results combining dietary guidelines with TPE. TPE has been associated with improvement in polyneuropathy, ichthyosis, ataxia, and cardiac involvement in most patients. Cranial nerve involvement (affecting vision, smell, and hearing) has not been affected by diet or TPE. Studies employing membrane differential ("cascade") filtration plasmapheresis have also been salutary.[138]

Other Storage Diseases

There is no evidence-based recommendation for use of TPE in Fabry's disease, Hunter's syndrome, Gaucher's disease, or X-linked adrenal leukodystrophy.

References

1. McLeod BC. Clinical applications of therapeutic apheresis. J Clin Apheresis 2000;15:1-5.
2. Smith JW, Weinstein R, Hillyer KL for the AABB Hemapheresis Committee. Therapeutic apheresis: A summary of current indication categories endorsed by the AABB and the American Society for Apheresis. Transfusion 2003;43:820-2.

3. Clark WF, Rock GA, Buskard N, et al. Therapeutic plasma exchange: An update from the Canadian apheresis group. Ann Intern Med 1999;131:453-62.
4. George JN. How I treat patients with thrombotic thrombocytopenic purpura—hemolytic uremic syndrome. Blood 2000;96:1223-9.
5. Moake JL. Thrombotic microangiopathies. N Engl J Med 2002;347:589-600.
6. Zheng XL, Kaufman RM, Goodnough LT, Sadler JE. Effect of plasma exchange on plasma ADAMTS13 metalloprotease activity, inhibitor level, and clinical outcome in patients with idiopathic and nonidiopathic thrombotic thrombocytopenic purpura. Blood 2004;103:4043-9.
7. Vesely SK, George JN, Lammle B, et al. ADAMTS13 activity in thrombotic thrombocytopenic purpura-hemolytic uremic syndrome: Relation to presenting features and clinical outcomes in a prospective cohort of 142 patients. Blood 2003;102:60-8.
8. George JN. Clinical course and long-term outcomes of thrombotic thrombocytopenic purpura. In: Sadler JE, Moake JL, Miyata T, George JN. Recent advances in thrombotic thrombocytopenic purpura. Hematology (Am Soc Hematol Educ Program) 2004:407-23.
9. Pereira A, Mazzara R, Monteagudo J, et al. Thrombotic thrombocytopenic purpura/hemolytic uremic syndrome: A multivariate analysis of factors predicting the response to plasma exhchange. Ann Hematol 1995;70:319-23.
10. Allford SL, Hunt BJ, Rose P, Machin SJ. Guidelines on the diagnosis and management of the thrombotic microangiopathic haemolytic anaemias. Br J Haematol 2003;120: 556-73.
11. Rock GA, Shumak KH, Buskard NA, et al. Comparison of plasma exhange and plasma infusion in the treatment of thrombotic thrombocytopenic purpura. N Engl J Med 1991;325:393-7.
12. Bandarenko N, Brecher ME. United States thrombotic thrombocytopenic purpura apheresis study group (US TTP ASG): Multicenter survey and retrospective analysis

of current efficacy of therapeutic plasma exchange. J Clin Apheresis 1998;13:133-41.

13. Zeigler Z and North American TTP Group. Cryoprecipitate poor plasma does not improve early response in primary adult thrombotic thrombocytopenic purpura. J Clin Apheresis 2001;16:19-22.

14. Yomtovian R, Niklinski W, Silver B, et al. Rituximab for chronic recurring thrombotic thrombocytopenic purpura: A case report and review of the literature. Br J Haematol 2004;124:787-95.

15. Crowther MA, Heddle N, Hayward CP, et al. Splenectomy done during hematologic remission to prevent relapse in patients with thrombotic thrombocytopenic purpura. Ann Intern Med 1996;125:294-6.

16. Melnyk AMS, Solez K, Kjellstrand CM. Adult hemolytic-uremic syndrome. Arch Intern Med 1995;155:2077-84.

17. Drew MJ. Therapeutic plasma exchange in hematologic diseases and dysproteinemias. In: McLeod BC, Price TH, Weinstein R, eds. Apheresis: Principles and practice. 2nd ed. Bethesda, MD: AABB Press, 2003:345-73.

18. Veyradier A, Obert B, Houllier A, et al. Specific von Willebrand factor-cleaving protease in thrombotic microangiopathies: A study of 111 cases. Blood 2001;98:1765-72.

19. Cattraan DC. Adult hemolytic-uremic syndrome: Successful treatment with plasmapheresis. Am J Kidney Dis 1984; 3:275-9.

20. George JN. The association of pregnancy with thrombotic thrombocytopenic purpura-hemolytic uremic syndrome. Curr Opin Hematol 2003;10:339-44.

21. Martin JN, Files JC, Blake PG, et al. Pregnancy complicated by preeclampsia-eclampsia with the syndrome of hemolysis, elevated liver enzymes, and low platelet count: How rapid is postpartum recovery? Obstet Gynecol 1990; 76:737-41.

22. Martin JN, Files JC, Blake PG, et al. Postpartum plasma exchange for atypical preeclampsia-eclampsia as HELLP (hemolysis, elevated liver enzymes, and low platelets) syndrome. Am J Obstet Gynecol 1995;172:1107-27.

23. Martin JN, Perry KG, Roberts WE, et al. Plasma exchange for preeclampsia: III. Immediate peripartal utilization for selected patients with HELLP syndrome. J Clin Apheresis 1994;9:162-5.

24. Martin JN, Perry KG, Roberts WE, et al. Plasma exchange for preeclampsia: II. Unsuccessful antepartum utilization for severe preeclampsia with or without HELLP syndrome. J Clin Apheresis 1994;9:155-61.

25. Kutti J, Wadenvik H, Safai-Kutti, et al. Successful treatment of refractory autoimmune haemolytic anemia by plasmapheresis. Scand J Haematol 1984;32:149-52.

26. Isbister JP, Biggs JC, Penny R. Experience with large volume plasmapheresis in malignant paraproteinaemia and immune disorders. Aust N Z J Med 1978;8:154-64.

27. Zaja F, Russo D, Fugo G, et al. Rituximab in a case of cold agglutinin disease. Br J Haematol 2001;115:232-4.

28. Silberstein LE, Berkman EM. Plasma exchange in autoimmune hemolytic anemia. J Clin Apheresis 1983;1:238-42.

29. Silva VA, Seder RH, Weintraub LR. Synchronization of plasma exchange and cyclophosphamide in severe and refractory autoimmune hemolytic anemia. J Clin Apheresis 1994;9:120-3.

30. Marder VJ, Nusbacher J, Anderson FW. One-year follow-up of plasma exchange therapy in 14 patients with idiopathic thrombocytopenic purpura. Transfusion 1981;21:291-8.

31. Jungi TW, Hydegger UE. Plasma exchange and intravenous immunoglobulin infusion: Effects on mononuclear phagocyte functions with potential implications for therapy. In: Rock G, ed. Apheresis. New York: Alan R. Liss, 1990:429-33.

32. Bussel JB, Saal S, Gordon B. Combined plasma exchange and intravenous gammaglobulin in the treatment of patients with refractory immune thrombocytopenic purpura. Transfusion 1988;28:38-41.

33. George JN, Woolf SH, Raskob GE, et al. Idiopathic thrombocytopenic purpura: A practice guideline developed by explicit methods for the American Society of Hematology. Blood 1996;88:3-40.

34. Brecher ME, Moore SB, Letendre L. Posttransfusion purpura: The therapeutic value of PlA1-negative platelets. Transfusion 1990;30:433-5.
35. Weisberg LJ, Linker CA. Prednisone therapy of posttransfusion purpura. Ann Intern Med 1984;100:76-7.
36. Chong BH, Cade J, Smith JA, Taboulis J. An unusual case of post-transfusion purpura: Good transient response to high dose immunoglobulin. Vox Sang 1986;51:182-4.
37. Cimo PL, Aster RH. Post-transfusion purpura: Successful treatment by exchange transfusion. N Engl J Med 1972; 287:290-2.
38. Slocombe GW, Newland AC, Colvin MP, et al. The role of intensive plasma exchange in the prevention and management of haemorrhage in patients with inhibitors to factor VIII. Br J Haematol 1981;47:577-85.
39. Bona RD, Pasquale DN, Kalish RI, et al. Porcine factor VIII and plasmapheresis in the management of hemophiliac patients with inhibitors. Am J Hematol 1986;21:201-7.
40. Pintado T, Taswell HF, Bowie EJW. Treatment of life-threatening hemorrhage due to acquired factor VIII inhibitor. Blood 1975;46:535-41.
41. Grima KM. Therapeutic apheresis in hematological and oncological diseases. J Clin Apheresis 2000;15:28-52.
42. Bloch KJ, Makl DG. Hyperviscosity syndromes associated with immunoglobulin abnormalities. Semin Hematol 1973;10:113-24.
43. Buskard NA, Glaton DAG, Goldman JM, et al. Plasma exchange in the long-term management of Waldenström's macroglobulinemia. CMAJ 1977;117:135-7.
44. Otaki AT. Plasma exchange v peritoneal dialysis for removing Bence Jones protein. Br Med J 1978;1397.
45. Solling K, Solling J. Clearances of Bence-Jones proteins during peritoneal dialysis or plasmapheresis in myelomatosis associated with renal failure. Contrib Nephrol 1988; 68:259-62.
46. Wahlin A, Lofvenberg E, Holm J. Improved survival in multiple myeloma with renal failure. Acta Med Scand 1987;221:205-9.

47. Misiani R, Tiraboschi G, Mingardi G, Meca G. Management of myeloma kidney: An anti-light-chain approach. Am J Kidney Dis 1987;10:28-33.
48. Zucchelli P, Pasquali S, Cagnoli L, Ferrari G. Controlled plasma exchange trial in acute renal failure due to multiple myeloma. Kidney Int 1988;33:1175-80.
49. Shehata N, Kouroukis C, Kelton JG. A review of randomized controlled trials using therapeutic apheresis. Transfus Med Rev 2002;16:200-29.
50. Berkman EM, Orlin JB. Use of plasmapheresis and partial plasma exchange in the management of patients with cryoglobulinemia. Transfusion 1980;20:171-8.
51. Geltner D, Kohn RW, Gorevic PD, et al. The effect of combination chemotherapy (steroids, immunosuppressives and plasmapheresis) on 5 mixed cryoglobulinemia patients with renal, neurologic and vascular involvement. Arthritis Rheum 1981;24:1121-7.
52. Winer JB. Guillain-Barré syndrome. J Clin Pathol:Mol Pathol 2001;54:381-5.
53. Raphael JC, Chevret S, Hughes RA, Annane D. Plasma exchange for Guillain-Barré syndrome. Cochrane Database Syst Rev 2002;(2):CD001798.
54. van der Meche FGA, Schmitz PIM and the Dutch Guillain-Barré Study Group. A randomized trial comparing intravenous immune globulin and plasma exchange in Guillain-Barré syndrome. N Engl J Med 1992;326:1123-9.
55. Bril V, Ilse WK, Pearce R, et al. Pilot trial of immunoglobulin versus plasma exchange in patients with Guillain-Barré syndrome. Neurology 1996;46:100-3.
56. Plasma Exchange/Sandoglobulin Guillain-Barré Syndrome Trial Group. Randomised trial of plasma exchange, intravenous immunoglobulin, and combined treatments in Guillain-Barré syndrome. Lancet 1997;349:225-30.
57. The Neuropathy Association, Medical Advisory Committee. Guidelines for the diagnosis and treatment of chronic inflammatory demyelinating polyneuropathy. J Peripher Nerv Syst 2003;8:282-4.

58. Bouchard C, Lacroix C, Plante V, et al. Clinicopathologic findings and prognosis of chronic inflammatory demyelinating polyneuropathy. Neurology 1999;52:498-503.

59. Yan WX, Archelos JJ, Hartung H-P, Pollard JD. P0 protein is a target antigen in chronic inflammatory demyelinating polyradiculoneuropathy. Ann Neurol 2001;50: 286-92.

60. Van Doorn PA, Ruts L. Treatment of chronic inflammatory demyelinating polyneuropathy. Curr Opin Neurol 2004;17:607-13.

61. Dyck PJ, Daube J, O'Brien P, et al. Plasma exchange in chronic inflammatory demyelinating polyradiculopathy. N Engl J Med 1986;314:461-5.

62. Hahn AF, Bolton CF, Pillay N, et al. Plasma-exchange therapy in chronic inflammatory demyelinating polyneuropathy. Brain 1996;119:1055-66.

63. Dispenzieri A, Kyle RA, Lacy MQ, et al. POEMS syndrome: Definitions and long-term outcome. Blood 2003; 101:2496-506.

64. Latov N. Evaluation and treatment of patients with neuropathy and monoclonal gammopathy. Semin Neurol 1994;14:118-22.

65. Comi G, Roveri L, Swan A, et al and the Inflammatory Neuropathy Cause and Treatment Group. A randomized controlled trial of intravenous immunoglobulin in IgM paraprotein associated demyelinating neuropathy. J Neurol 2002;249:1370-7.

66. Dyck PJ, Low PA, Windebank AJ, et al. Plasma exchange in polyneuropathy associated with monoclonal gammopathy of undetermined significance. N Engl J Med 1991; 325:1482-6.

67. Pascuzzi RM. Myasthenia gravis and Lambert-Eaton syndrome. Ther Apheresis 2002;6:57-68.

68. Vincent A, Rothwell P. Myasthenia gravis. Autoimmunity 2004;37:317-9.

69. Juel VC, Massey JM. Autoimmune myasthenia gravis: Recommendations for treatment and immunologic modulation. Curr Treat Options Neurol 2005;7:3-14.

70. Dau PC, Lindstrom JM, Cassel CK, et al. Plasmapheresis and immunosuppressive drug therapy in myasthenia gravis. N Engl J Med 1977;297:1134-40.
71. Mahalati K, Dawson RB, Collins JO, Mayer RF. Predictable recovery from myasthenia gravis crisis with plasma exchange: Thirty-six cases and review of current management. J Clin Apheresis 1999;14:1-8.
72. Qureshi AI, Choundry MA, Akbar MS, et al. Plasma exchange versus intravenous immunoglobulin treatment in myasthenic crisis. Neurology 1999;52:629-32.
73. Gajdos P, Chevret S, Clair B, et al for the Myasthenia Gravis Clinical Study Group. Clinical trial of plasma exchange and high-dose intravenous immunoglobulin in myasthenia gravis. Ann Neurol 1997;41:789-96.
74. Sanders DB. Lambert-Eaton myasthenic syndrome: Diagnosis and treatment. Ann N Y Acad Sci 2003;998:500-8.
75. Storch MK, Piddlesden S, Haltia M, et al. Multiple sclerosis: In situ evidence for antibody- and complement-mediated demyelination. Ann Neurol 1998;43:465-7.
76. Berger T, Rubner P, Schautzer F, et al. Antimyelin antibodies as a predictor of clinically definite multiple sclerosis after a first demyelinating event. N Engl J Med 2003; 349:139-45.
77. Transverse Myelitis Consortium Working Group. Proposed diagnostic criteria and nosology of acute transverse myelitis. Neurology 2002;59:499-505.
78. Zhang J, Hutton G. Role of magnetic resonance imaging and immunotherapy in treating multiple sclerosis. Annu Rev Med 2005;56:273-302.
79. Weiner HL, Dau PC, Khatri BO, et al. Double-blind study of true vs. sham plasma exchange in patients treated with immunosuppression for acute attacks of multiple sclerosis. Neurology 1989;39:1143-9.
80. The Canadian Cooperative Multiple Sclerosis Study Group. The Canadian cooperative trial of cyclophosphamide and plasma exchange in progressive multiple sclerosis. Lancet 1991;337:441-6.
81. Weinshenker BG, O'Brien PC, Petterson TM, et al. A randomized trial of plasma exchange in acute central nervous

system inflammatory demyelinating disease. Ann Neurol 1999;46:878-86.

82. Koerner C, Wieland B, Richter W, Meinck H-M. Stiff-person syndromes: Motor cortex hyperexcitability correlates with anti-GAD autoimmunity. Neurology 2004;62:1357-62.

83. Dalakas MC, Fujii M, Li M, McElroy B. The clinical spectrum of anti-GAD antibody-positive patients with stiff-person syndrome. Neurology 2000;55:1531-5.

84. Griswold W, Drlicek M. Paraneoplastic neuropathy. Curr Opin Neurol 1999;12:617-25.

85. Moll JWB, Vecht ChJ. Immune diagnosis of paraneoplastic neurological disease. Clin Neurol Neurosurg 1995; 97:71-81.

86. Darnell RB, Posner JB. Paraneoplastic syndromes involving the nervous system. N Engl J Med 2003;349:1543-54.

87. Das A, Hochberg FH, McNelis S. A review of the therapy of paraneoplastic neurologic syndromes. J Neurooncol 1999;41:181-94.

88. Hudson BG, Tryggvason K, Sundaramoorthy M, Neilson EG. Alport's syndrome, Goodpasture's syndrome, and type IV collagen. N Engl J Med 2003;348:2543-56.

89. Johnson JP, Moore J, Austin HA, et al. Therapy of anti-glomerular basement antibody disease: Analysis of prognostic significance of clinical, pathologic and treatment factors. Medicine (Baltimore) 1985;64:219-27.

90. Levy JB, Turner AN, Rees AJ, Pusey CD. Long-term outcome of anti-glomerular basement membrane antibody disease treated with plasma exchange and immunosuppression. Ann Intern Med 2001;134:1033-42.

91. Glockner WM, Sieberth HG, Wichmann HE, et al. Plasma exchange and immunosuppression in rapidly progressive glomerulonephritis: A controlled, multicenter study. Clin Nephrol 1988;29:1-8.

92. Cole E, Cattran D, Magil A, et al. A prospective randomized trial of plasma exchange as additive therapy in idiopathic crescentic glomerulonephritis. The Canadian Apheresis Study Group. Am J Kidney Dis 1992;20:261-9.

93. Benchimol C. Focal segmental glomerulosclerosis: Pathogenesis and treatment. Curr Opin Pediatr 2003;15: 171-80.

94. Savin VJ, Sharma R, Sharma M, et al. Circulating factor associated with increased glomerular permeability to albumin in recurrent focal segmental glomerulosclerosis. N Engl J Med 1996;334:878-83.

95. Davenport RD. Apheresis treatment of recurrent focal segmental glomerulosclerosis after kidney transplantation: Re-analysis of published case-reports and case-series. J Clin Apheresis 2001;16:175-8.

96. Racusen LC, Colvin RB, Solez K, et al. Antibody-mediated rejection criteria—an addition to the Banff '97 classification of renal allograft rejection. Am J Transplant 2003; 3:708-14.

97. Kirubakaran MG, Disney AP, Norman J, et al. A controlled trial of plasmapheresis in the treatment of renal allograft rejection. Transplantation 1981;32:164-5.

98. Allen NH, Dyer P, Geoghegan T, et al. Plasma exchange in acute renal allograft rejection: A controlled trial. Transplantation 1983;35:425-8.

99. Bonomini V, Vangelista A, Frasca GM, et al. Effects of plasmapheresis in renal transplant rejection. A controlled trial. Trans Am Soc Artif Intern Organs 1985;31:698-703.

100. Blake P, Sutton D, Cardella CJ. Plasma exchange in acute renal transplant rejection. Prog Clin Biol Res 1990;337: 249-52.

101. Montgomery RA, Zachary AA, Racusen LC, et al. Plasmapheresis and intravenous immune globulin provides effective rescue therapy for refractory humoral rejection and allows kidneys to be successfully transplanted into crossmatch-positive recipients. Transplantation 2000;70:887-95.

102. Takahashi K, Saito K, Takahara S, et al and the Japanese ABO-incompatible Kidney Transplantation Committee. Excellent long-term outcome of ABO-incompatible living donor kidney transplantation in Japan. Am J Transplant 2004;4:1089-96.

103. Sonnenday CJ, Warren DS, Cooper M, et al. Plasmapheresis, CMV hyperimmune globulin, and anti-CD20 al-

low ABO-incompatible renal transplantation without splenectomy. Am J Transplant 2004;4:1315-22.

104. Winters JL, Gloor JM, Pineda AA, et al. Plasma exchange conditioning for ABO-incompatible renal transplantation. J Clin Apheresis 2004;19:79-85.

105. Robinson JA, Radvany RM, Mullen MG, Garrity ER Jr. Plasmapheresis followed by intravenous immunoglobulin in presensitized patients awaiting thoracic organ transplantation. Ther Apher 1997;1:147-51.

106. West LJ, Pollock-Barziv SM, Dipchand AI, et al. ABO-incompatible heart transplantation in infants. N Engl J Med 2001;344:793-800.

107. Renard TH, Andrews WS. An approach to ABO-incompatible liver transplantation in children. Transplantation 1992;53:116-21.

108. Kawagishi N, Ohkohchi N, Fujimori K, et al. Indications and efficacy of apheresis for liver transplant recipients: Experience of 16 cases in 34 living-related liver transplants. Transplant Proc 2000;32:2111-3.

109. Monteiro I, McLoughlin LM, Fisher A, et al. Rituximab with plasmapheresis and splenectomy in ABO-incompatible liver transplantation. Transplantation 2003;76:1648-9.

110. Mandal AK, King KE, Humphreys SL, et al. Plasmapheresis: An effective therapy for primary allograft nonfunction after liver transplantation. Transplantation 2000;70:216-20.

111. Skerrett D, Mor E, Curtiss S, Mohandas K. Plasmapheresis in primary dysfunction of hepatic transplants. J Clin Apheresis 1996;11:10-3.

112. Reeves GEM. Update on the immunology, diagnosis and management of systemic lupus erythematosus. Intern Med J 2004;34:338-47.

113. Wei N, Klippel JH, Huston DP, et al. Randomised trial of plasma exchange in mild systemic lupus erythematosus. Lancet 1983;i:17-22.

114. Bambauer R, Schwarze U, Schiel R. Cyclosporin A and therapeutic plasma exchange in the treatment of severe systemic lupus erythematosus. Artif Organs 2000;24: 852-6.

111

115. Lewis EJ, Hunsicker LG, Lan SP, et al. A controlled trial of plasmapheresis therapy in severe lupus nephritis. The Lupus Nephritis Collaborative Study Group. N Engl J Med 1992;326:1373-9.

116. Levine JS, Branch DW, Rauch J. The antiphospholipid syndrome. N Engl J Med 2002;346:752-63.

117. Flamholz R, Tran T, Grad GI, et al. Therapeutic plasma exchange for the acute management of the catastrophic antiphospholipid syndrome: β2-glycoprotein I antibodies as a marker of response to therapy. J Clin Apheresis 1999;14:171-6.

118. Atherson RA, Cervera R, Piette J-C, et al. Catastrophic antiphospholipid syndrome: Clinical and laboratory features of 50 patients. Medicine 1998;77:195-207.

119. Bacon PA. The spectrum of Wegener's granulomatosis and disease relapse. N Engl J Med 2005;352:330-2.

120. Guillevin L, Pagnoux C. Indications of plasma exchange for systemic vasculitides. Ther Apher Dial 2003;7:155-60.

121. Hassanein TI, Wahlstrom E, Zamora JU, Van Thiel DH. Conventional care of fulminant hepatic failure: Medical and surgical aspects. Ther Apheresis 1997;1:33-7.

122. Kaplan AA, Epstein M. Extracorporeal blood purification in the management of patients with hepatic failure. Semin Nephrol 1997;17:576-82.

123. Redeker AG, Yamahiro HS. Controlled trial of exchange-transfusion therapy in fulminant hepatitis. Lancet 1973;i:3-6.

124. Lepore MJ, Stutman LJ, Bonanno CA, et al. Plasmapheresis with plasma exchange in hepatic coma. Arch Intern Med 1972;129:900-7.

125. Buckner CD, Clift RA, Volwiler W, et al. Plasma exchange in patients with fulminant hepatic failure. Arch Intern Med 1973;132:487-92.

126. Kondrup J, Almdal T, Vilstrup H, Tygstrup N. High volume plasma exchange in fulminant hepatic failure. Int J Artif Organs 1992;15:669-76.

127. Larsen FS, Hansen BA, Jorgensen LG, et al. High-volume plasmapheresis and acute liver transplantation in fulminant hepatic failure. Transplant Proc 1994;26:1788.

128. Singer AL, Olthoff KM, Kim H, et al. Role of plasma-pheresis in the management of acute hepatic failure in children. Ann Surg 2001;234:418-24.

129. Kiss JE, Berman D, van Thiel D. Effective removal of copper by plasma exchange in fulminant Wilson's disease. Transfusion 1998;38:327-31.

130. Kamochi M, Aibara K, Nakata K, et al. Profound ionized hypomagnesemia induced by therapeutic plasma exchange in liver failure patients. Transfusion 2002;42:1598-602.

131. Litovitz TL, Klein-Schwartz W, Dyer KS, et al. 1997 report of the American Association of Poison Control Centers toxic exposure surveillance system. Am J Emerg Med 1998;16:443-97.

132. Winters JL, Pineda AA, McLeod BC, Grima KM. Therapeutic apheresis in renal and metabolic diseases. J Clin Apheresis 2000;15:53-73.

133. Szczepiorkowski Z. TPE in renal, rheumatic, and miscellaneous disorders. In: McLeod BC, Price TH, Weinstein R, eds. Apheresis: Principles and practice. 2nd ed. Bethesda, MD: AABB Press, 2003:375-409.

134. Piqueras J, Duran-Suarez JR, Massuet L, et al. Mushroom poisoning: Therapeutic apheresis or forced diuresis. Transfusion 1987;27:116-7.

135. Finestone AJ, Berman R, Widner B. Thioctic acid treatment of acute mushroom poisoning. Penn Med 1972;75:49-51.

136. Trujillo MH, Guerrero J, Fragachan C, et al. Pharmacologic antidotes in critical care medicine: A practical guide for drug administration. Crit Care Med 1998;26:377-91.

137. Gibberd FB, Billimoria JD, Page NGR, Retsas S. Heredopathia atactica polyneuritiformis (Refsum's disease) treated by diet and plasma-exchange. Lancet 1979;i:575-8.

138. Siegmund JB, Meier H, Hoppmann I, Gutsche H-U. Cascade filtration in Refsum's disease. Nephrol Dial Transplant 1995;10:117-9.

RED CELL EXCHANGE

Introduction

Red cell exchange (RCE) is the selective removal of a patient's red cells and the simultaneous replacement with donor red cells. Most applications of RCE are in the treatment of sickle cell disease (SCD).[1]

Automated Red Cell Exchange

Standard Technique

Current apheresis instruments, such as the Spectra (Gambro BCT, Lakewood, CO), utilize fully automated, integral, programmable, computerized control systems. When a patient's height, weight, gender, and hematocrit levels are entered, the instrument calculates total blood volume (TBV) and red cell volume (RCV). Other information required for RCE includes the desired postprocedure hematocrit, the hematocrit of the Red Blood Cell (RBC) units to be infused, and the desired fraction of cells remaining (FCR) at the end of the procedure. On the basis of these parameters, the instrument calculates the appropriate red cell volumes to be removed and replaced. The whole blood-to-anticoagulant ratio (AC ratio) is preset at 13:1; however, it can be adjusted manually if required.

Generally an exchange equivalent to a little over one patient RCV will remove approximately 70% of the patient's own red cells, leaving an FCR of about 30%. A two-volume exchange will deplete about 90% of red cells, leaving an FCR of 10%. When RCE is planned for SCD, it is important to know the history of any recent blood transfusion because that will influence the quantity of red cells that needs to be exchanged. A recent hemoglobin electrophoresis result is the most useful guide. If a patient has not been transfused within the past 2 months, it can be assumed that the hemoglobin S (HbS) level is 100%. The goal is often to reduce the HbS level to 30%. Thus, if the pretreatment HbS is 100%, the FCR programmed into the machine should be 30%. The FCR can be adjusted appropriately if pretreatment HbS is thought to be substantially less than 100% or if a post-RCE HbS less than 30% is desired. Using entries for the patient's hematocrit, height, and weight, the apheresis instrument will calculate the exact quantity of red cells needed. However, the instrument calculation is often not available at the time when blood must be ordered for the procedure. Thus, a physician may have to estimate the required number of RBC units. A simple approach begins with calculating the patient's TBV based on a 70-mL/kg formula. The patient's RCV can then be calculated by multiplying TBV times the hematocrit divided by 100. For example, TBV in a 50-kg patient is 3500 mL; if the hematocrit is 20%, the RCV is calculated as $3500 \times (20/100) = 700$ mL. Each RBC unit contains approximately 180 mL of red cells (even though the volume of an AS RBC unit may be higher: eg, ~330 mL with a hematocrit of 55%). Thus for a one-volume exchange (ie, 30% FCR), this patient will require about 700 mL of red cells; this is equivalent to $700/180 = 3.9$ units, which would be rounded up to 4 RBC units. To increase the hematocrit during the exchange would require roughly one additional unit for each 3% increase desired. For example, to increase this patient's hematocrit from 20% to 23% would require one more unit. Thus, if this is the goal, the physician should order 5 RBC units for RCE.

RBC units given during RCE should be leukocyte reduced to prevent febrile nonhemolytic transfusion reactions because, if there is a reaction, the procedure must be halted until investigation is complete. Ideally, donor RBC units should also be tested for sickle cell trait.

In smaller children (body weight < 20 kg) or patients with severe anemia (hematocrit <18%), there is concern about the removal of >15% of patient's red cell mass in the machine during RCE. This can cause sudden hypoxemia in an anemic patient. To circumvent this problem in small or anemic patients, the apheresis machine can be primed with blood instead of normal saline, so that donor blood (instead of normal saline) enters the return line when patient blood is drawn into the machine. This will prevent a sudden decrease in red cell mass in the patient's circulation. This modification to the usual procedure is described in greater detail in the section on Pediatric Therapeutic Apheresis.

Some patients who are chronically exposed to donor red cells will make alloantibodies. Antigens in the Rh and Kell systems are the most antigenic; therefore, antibodies in these systems tend to develop first in sickle cell patients who will make antibodies.[2] Some centers make it a policy to transfuse SCD patients with red cells that are matched for the patient's Rh and Kell antigens (partial phenotypic match) so that these common alloantibodies can be avoided. This requires extra effort to find antigen-negative units for patients who have not formed antibodies, but often obviates the need for repeated antibody identification procedures.

Isovolemic Hemodilution

Traditional RCE has been modified in some centers for improved efficacy. Isovolemic hemodilution RCE (IHD-RCE) is performed in two steps, each of which must be programmed separately in the apheresis instrument. During the IHD step, patient red cells are removed and replaced with normal saline (150-300 mL) to an extent expected to decrease the hematocrit by 3% to 6%. The quantity of red cells to be removed and replaced in this way depends on the patient's hematocrit and blood volume. The hematocrit at the end of the IHD step should not be <20%; therefore, IHD-RCE should not be performed if the baseline hematocrit is <23%. During the second step, routine RCE is performed with the end hematocrit specified at or above that of baseline. During the IHD phase, HbS-containing red cells are removed with no admixture of donor red cells, thus allowing for more efficient depletion of HbS.[3] IHD-RCE requires about 15 to 20 minutes longer procedure time than traditional RCE; however, the advantages outweigh this extra time, as described below.

Urgent Need

Indications for acute RCE include certain complications of SCD, red cells affected by chemical poisoning, and severe protozoal diseases, as discussed below. In the case of urgent exchange for stroke or acute chest syndrome, where there is an immediate need for red cells with unimpaired oxygen-carrying capacity, it may be advantageous to use the freshest available red cells (ideally <7 days old) so that the 2,3-diphosphoglycerate content will be near normal and oxygen delivery will be optimal.[4] Also, to prevent delay, an institutional requirement for partial phenotype matching can be waived for an urgent RCE.

Side Effects

Transfusion reactions can occur during RCE. Premedication with acetaminophen or diphenhydramine can be given to prevent febrile nonhemolytic or allergic reactions, respectively, in patients with a history of reactions. Citrate reactions may also be noted during RCE and may include nausea, vomiting, and/or abdominal cramps as well as acral and perioral paresthesias, muscle cramps, and, occasionally, frank tetany. The preset AC ratio is 13:1. A higher AC ratio (eg, between 14:1 and 15:1) and/or calcium supplementation can be used for a patient having repeated citrate reactions. Thrombocytosis (platelet count >400,000/μL) is common among SCD patients,[5] and their platelets may be more likely to clump in the instrument with a preset AC ratio of 13:1. This platelet clumping tendency could be combated by lowering the AC ratio (eg, between 11:1 and 12:1) to infuse more anticoagulant; however, this may promote citrate reactions. Another approach to preventing platelet clumping without giving additional anticoagulant is to give 325 mg aspirin on the day of RCE to eligible patients whose platelet counts exceed 300,000/μL.

Monitoring

Pre- and postprocedure complete blood counts and hemoglobin electrophoreses should be performed to monitor the outcome of RCE. Patients experiencing repeated citrate reactions may also have ionized calcium levels drawn during the procedure to plan for calcium supplementation. Ferritin levels should be measured at 3- to 6-month intervals to monitor iron stores in patients on maintenance RCE.

Vascular Access

Peripheral venous access should be employed for RCE whenever possible because the complication rate is lower; specifically, the risk of infection is minimal. Generally, a 16- to 18-gauge cannula or back-eye needle is placed for blood withdrawal, while a smaller (19- to 20-gauge) device can be used for return if necessary. In older children and adults, antecubital veins are often suitable for withdrawal and return. For patients without good peripheral veins, a temporary dual-lumen venous catheter can be placed in a femoral vein for access. In most cases, because RCE for SCD will not be needed again for at least a month, the catheter can be removed when the procedure is finished.

Implantable ports are catheters placed completely under the skin; therefore, the risk of infection is extremely low. The distal (upstream) end of the catheter is attached to a small metal "drum" or reservoir, which has a membrane on one side for needle access. The entire device is surgically inserted just below the clavicle, with the drum membrane lying immediately below the skin and the catheter running subcutaneously from the drum into the subclavian vein. Access for apheresis is obtained with a special needle that is pushed through both skin and membrane into the reservoir inside the drum. Implantable ports such as the Vortex (Horizon Medical Products, Atlanta, GA) are available in different lengths and gauges with either one or two lumens. To perform RCE in a patient with a single-lumen device, blood can be withdrawn from the port and returned through a peripheral vein, or vice versa. The complexity of accessing implantable ports plus the lack of experience with them among apheresis technicians has limited their popularity for therapeutic apheresis.

Occasionally an arteriovenous fistula can be used for long-term RCE.[6] Such fistulas are placed routinely for dialysis in renal failure patients who are hypocoagulable. However, use of such fistulas in SCD patients is uncommon because of concern about a high risk of occlusion.

Indications

Clinical indications for RCE that have been rated by AABB[7] and the American Society for Apheresis (ASFA)[8] are listed in Table 11.

Sickle Cell Disease

Because patients with SCD are homozygous for HbS, they are prone to various complications related to intravascular red cell sickling, and their median survival age is 53 years.[9] Morbidity and mortality are due to hemolytic anemia, infections, large vessel thrombosis, occlusions in the microvasculature, and resultant chronic organ damage. RCE is indicated in various SCD crises. Emergent RCE is generally indicated for patients presenting with acute chest syndrome, stroke, retinal infarction, or persistent priapism not responding to conservative management after 24 hours and, occasionally, repeated intractable pain crises that are resistant to standard management. In addition, RCE may be performed during pregnancy and before prolonged general anesthesia under certain circumstances.

Neurologic Complications

The most devastating SCD complications are central nervous system (CNS) events. About 5% to 7% of children suffer an ischemic

Table 11. Indications for Red Blood Cell Exchange (ASFA/AABB Guidelines)[7,8]

- Sickle cell disease (Category I)
  - Acute chest syndrome
  - Stroke
  - Persistent priapism
  - Rarely perioperative in selected cases
  - Intractable pain crisis resistant to standard management

- Protozoal disease (Category III)
  - Malaria
  - Babesiosis

- Mismatched blood transfusion (not rated)
  - Rh-negative patient received substantial amount of Rh-positive blood
  - ABO-mismatched marrow transplantation
  - Passenger lymphocyte syndrome

- Intoxication (not rated)
  - CO poisoning
  - Methemoglobinemia

---

stroke, the incidence being 0.6 per 100 patient years.[10] The mortality for a first childhood stroke in recent years has been low (<2%), and the majority of patients (>60%) recover gross function.[11] Unfortunately, about two-thirds will have another CNS event within 3 years if measures are not taken to maintain HbS values at a safe level (<30%). About one-third of initial strokes in SCD occur in adults; most of these are hemorrhagic, and mortality is high (~50%).[11]

Ischemic stroke and transient ischemic attacks are usually secondary to intracranial arteriopathy involving the terminal internal carotid, the proximal middle cerebral, or the anterior cerebral arteries. The arterial changes can be detected by transcranial Doppler ultrasound or magnetic resonance angiography.[12] SCD patients are also at risk for other CNS events including cavernous sinus thrombosis, reversible posterior leukoencephalopathy, and acute demyelination.[12] Predisposing factors for CNS events include severe anemia, granulocytosis, adhesion of abnormal sickle cells to endothelial cells resulting from expression of VCAM-1 and ICAM-1, and thrombocytosis, which is present in the majority of patients.[13] The most common presentation is hemiparesis; however, aphasia, seizures, coma, and monoparesis are also seen.[10]

Immediate Transfusion Management: Following an acute CNS event, the goal is to improve cerebral oxygenation with oxygen supplementation (peripheral saturation >96% using pulse oximetry) and to maintain hydration. Red cell transfusion is recommended to improve anemia and lower HbS levels, both to prevent progression and to promote healing in the lesion, but there is no consensus regarding whether simple red cell transfusion or urgent RCE within a few hours of presentation is preferable. The goal of either form of red cell transfusion therapy is to reduce HbS to <30% while avoiding the increased blood viscosity and diminished CNS blood flow that could result from raising the hematocrit above 30%. Simple transfusion can be performed at any hospital; however, in the majority of patients, the volume that can be transfused without raising the hematocrit above 30% will not dilute the HbS level to the desired level. On the other hand, RCE performed urgently can achieve both goals, ie, decrease HbS to <30% while avoiding hyperviscosity by maintaining hematocrit <30% or near the patient's baseline value. Therefore, in patients with stroke, centers with an apheresis service often opt for an urgent RCE. Sometimes patients who receive red cell transfusions at one hospital are referred to another for RCE. In this case, it is useful to know how many units were transfused, because an RCE with a higher FCR (eg, 50% vs 30%) will require fewer RBC units.

Long-Term Transfusion Management: Because of the high incidence of recurrence,[14] children who have had a stroke are customarily put on a red cell transfusion regimen that will maintain HbS <30% for the first 3 to 4 years. This strategy has reduced the recurrence of CNS events to <10%. After 3 to 4 years, a lower risk of recurrent stroke can be realized by maintaining

HbS at <50%, possibly indefinitely or at least until new therapy emerges.[4]

These HbS goals can be achieved in two ways. One is chronic transfusion therapy (CTT). Small children with poor venous access usually undergo CTT during which they receive 10 to 15 mL/kg of red cells every 3 to 4 weeks. CTT can maintain the desired HbS values in most patients. It provides HbA-containing cells and suppresses the patient's marrow so that it produces fewer HbS-containing cells. The advantages of CTT are the single venous access requirement and the ability to carry out the treatment at any hospital. Disadvantages include frequent day-long visits to the hospital and inevitable iron overload requiring unpleasant chelation therapy.

The alternative is RCE. Patients who have adequate dual venous access can undergo maintenance RCE. Compared with CTT, the advantages of RCE include prevention of iron overload (because red cells removed from the patient's circulation will compensate to a great extent for those transfused), a shorter hospital visit (half a day) because RCE is much faster (~90 minutes) than transfusion of several units of blood (~2 hours/unit), and a slightly increased interval between procedures (4-5 weeks). Disadvantages of RCE procedures are the expense and the increased RBC unit requirement, which translates into more donor exposures. Additionally, the requirement for dual venous access can be technically challenging, especially in smaller children. It may be desirable to have pediatric personnel establish venous access before the apheresis technician arrives; lines can then be kept patent by normal saline infusion.

IHD-RCE (described above) can be used in place of traditional RCE for patients undergoing long-term RCE and appears to have several advantages in this context. These include more efficient lowering of HbS-containing cells during the IHD phase, a reduction by 1 to 2 units per procedure in the quantity of red cells required, which translates into fewer donor exposures, and an increased interval between procedures: ie, 7 to 8 weeks for IHD-RCE vs 4 to 5 weeks for standard RCE.[3] A decreased frequency of treatment will reduce cost, inconvenience, and time away from school or work.

The targeted post-RCE hematocrit can be increased gradually over several months to years from a baseline of 25% to 27% to 30%, and then to 32%. This incremental increase allows the patient's vasculature to adjust to a higher hematocrit and ultimately improves energy and physical activity levels.[3]

Primary Stroke Prevention: Recent studies indicate that measurement of cerebral blood flow velocity and vascular flow patterns by transcranial Doppler ultrasonography can identify SCD patients at high risk for ischemic stroke. The Stroke Prevention Trial in Sickle Cell Anemia (STOP) study demonstrated that CTT reduces the occurrence of first stroke in children with an elevated cerebral blood flow velocity detected in this way.[15] The STOPII trial that began in 2000 was halted 2 years early because of recurrence of stroke and worsening of risk for stroke parameters.[16]

Marrow transplantation may be offered to patients with HLA-matched siblings. Nietert et al[17] compared outcomes of marrow transplantation with periodic red cell transfusion as a basis for making treatment recommendations for patients at high risk for ischemic stroke. Their analysis showed that marrow transplantation has no significant advantage over CTT and, therefore, cannot be considered the optimal strategy for these patients at this time.

Acute Chest Syndrome

Acute chest syndrome (ACS) is a serious complication of SCD that carries mortality rates of about 1% in children and 4% in adults.[18] ACS is characterized by clinical or radiographic evidence of new or progressive pulmonary disease. Its etiology is often multifactorial. The clinical course ranges from a self-limited illness to acute respiratory failure requiring mechanical ventilation, but in general its severity differs greatly between young children and adults. ACS in children is generally mild and most likely is caused by infection. In contrast, adults seem to suffer more from pulmonary sequestration events, which lead to severe hypoxia, prolonged hospitalizations, and the higher death rate. Recurrent episodes of ACS may also cause chronic lung disease and premature death.[19]

Optimal management includes hydration, antibiotics, supplemental oxygen, and red cell therapy.[4] There is no randomized study to determine whether RCE or simple transfusion is preferable. The choice between these two alternatives often depends on the hemoglobin level and the severity of the patient's illness.[20] Diffuse bilateral pulmonary infiltrates, hypoxia, and a presenting hematocrit that is lower than baseline have been found to correlate with a worse prognosis.[18] A sudden decrease in the hematocrit from baseline (eg, to <18%) suggests that the episode of ACS involves sequestration of sickled red cells in the pulmonary vasculature. These clinical features are useful in the selection of patients for red cell therapy. Simple transfusion is technically easier as well as more feasible at smaller hospitals. However, aggressive transfusion is required to decrease HbS to <30%. This in turn may increase the hematocrit significantly above baseline. Once sickled cells trapped in the lung undergo unsickling, they are released into the circulation. This may raise the hematocrit further, thus increasing the risk of a CNS event due to hyperviscosity. In such patients, therefore, RCE appears to be a better choice to lower the HbS level, correct anemia, and improve oxygen transport.

Ideally the apheresis service should be alerted as soon as a diagnosis of ACS is suspected so that arrangements can be made for urgent RCE. Because these patients are already hypoxemic and RCE replaces nearly 70% of circulating red cells with donor cells, it may be desirable to use relatively fresh red cells (ideally, <10 days old) in this circumstance. The fresher cells also provide immediate optimal oxygen-carrying capacity in the transfused red cells.[21] Restoration of normal oxygen-carrying capacity in red cells nearer the end of their storage life may take 12 to 24 hours after transfusion. If partial phenotype matching is practiced, the requirement should be waived in favor of fresher red cells. While results of RCE are generally dramatic, with rapid normalization of arterial oxygen saturation, attendant infiltrates may take days to resolve.

Priapism

Priapism is another serious complication encountered in about 40% of adult males and about 6% of preadolescent males with SCD.[22] Conservative management of priapism includes hydration, alkalinization, and simple transfusion. However, a severe episode that does not respond within 24 hours should be treated urgently with RCE to avoid the necessity for surgical intervention (aspiration and irrigation of corpora cavernosa, and vascular shunting). Both persistent priapism and surgical intervention can lead to impotence.[23] The goal of RCE is to reduce HbS to <30% while raising the hematocrit no higher than 30%. The ASPEN syndrome (*A*ssociation of *S*ickle cell disease, *P*riapism, *E*xchange transfusion, and *N*eurologic events) has been described in these patients.[24] Severe headache is generally the first symptom and is followed by lethargy, seizures, and stroke. Neurologic events can occur up to 2 weeks after RCE. The ASPEN syndrome is attributed to sudden release of unsickled red cells from the corpora cavernosa into the circulation, raising the hematocrit above 36%. It may also be related to release of vasoactive substances during penile detumescence. The higher hematocrit could lead to hyperviscosity, while the vasoactive materials could exacerbate cerebral hypoxia. As noted above, similar complications can occur after RCE in ACS as well.

Pregnancy

SCD patients are at higher risk for morbidity and mortality during pregnancy. Toxemia, intrauterine growth retardation, pre-eclampsia, and premature labor and delivery are possible complications that place both mother and fetus at risk. Additionally, common SCD-related problems may be exacerbated by pregnancy. There is no current consensus about transfusion protocol in pregnant patients with SCD. At one extreme is a UK recommendation for universal RCE beginning at 28 weeks of gestation and earlier prophylactic transfusion therapy for women whose obstetric or hematologic history suggests a high risk of complications.[25] On the other hand, US institutions seldom use prophylactic transfusion therapy. Assessments of fetal and maternal hemodynamics have demonstrated negligible changes during and after RCE in pregnant patients.[26]

Perioperative Management

Both surgery and anesthesia may trigger complications such as ACS, renal failure, stroke, and pain crisis.[27,28] In the past, SCD patients requiring surgical intervention were at increased risk for developing crisis because conditions that promote sickling (such as hypoxia, dehydration, and electrolyte abnormalities) were common during anesthesia. Close monitoring and improved techniques during anesthesia have lessened the risk of intraoperative SCD-related complications. Currently there is no consensus regarding routine preoperative transfusion therapy. Therefore, each case must be individually assessed for level of risk. Preexisting hepatic, cardiac, pulmonary, renal, and neurologic problems must be considered along with the expected duration of anesthesia, the expected amount of blood loss, as well as any history of SCD complications. Similarly, the type of surgery (eg, cardiopulmonary bypass, neurosurgery, and retinal and vitreous surgery) may also warrant consideration of transfusion therapy.[29,30] If a patient is considered at high risk, the hematocrit should be increased to close to 30% and HbS decreased to <30% shortly before surgery. Simple red cell transfusion can achieve the hematocrit goal but not the HbS goal when surgery must be performed urgently; however, both goals can be met easily by RCE.

Thalassemia

Chronic transfusion is the mainstay of therapy for patients with beta thalassemia. But, as in SCD, it inevitably produces iron overloading. In one study, patients with thalassemia were randomly assigned to a conventional transfusion regimen or RCE. RCE significantly increased the transfusion interval by 43% (from 35.7 days to 51 days), decreased red cell requirement by 30% (from 0.41 mL/kg/day to 0.29 mL/kg/day), and decreased iron loading (as judged by ferritin levels) when compared to simple transfusion.[31]

Protozoal Diseases

RCE can be used to remove red cells infected with protozoal parasites. Such therapy is recommended for only two protozoal infections, namely, malaria and babesiosis.

Malaria

Indications for RCE in malaria include infection with drug-resistant strains or severe *Plasmodium falciparum* malaria with hyperparasitemia. The World Health Organization classification defines "severe or complicated malaria" as those cases presenting with various combinations of the following manifestations: 1) hyperparasitemia (>5%), 2) encephalopathy or cerebral malaria, 3) jaundice (bilirubin >2.5 mg/dL), 4) severe anemia (hematocrit <20%), 5) acute renal failure (creatinine >3 mg/dL), 6) respiratory distress, 7) hypoglycemia (glucose <40 mg/dL), 8) disseminated intravascular coagulation, and 9) circulatory collapse and shock.[32]

Babesiosis

American babesiosis is generally a subclinical or mild disease. However, splenectomized or immunocompromised patients are at risk for a severe disease, although they usually respond well to antibiotic therapy. Rarely, refractory babesiosis patients with high parasitemia (>20%) have responded well to RCE as an adjunct therapy. Unlike the situation in malaria, there is no extraerythrocytic reservoir of babesia, and, therefore, RCE is very effective in lowering parasite load.[33]

RCE Plan for Protozoal Diseases

In either clinical condition, a 1.5 to 2 RCV exchange (FCR of 10-20%) should be performed to reduce parasitemia. The hematocrit should be raised to 35% to correct anemia and improve oxygenation. Pre- and postprocedure parasite counts should be performed to assess the outcome of the procedure. A second RCE may be needed for patients with very high initial parasitemia (>30%).

Mismatched Red Cell Transfusion

Rarely, it is necessary to transfuse an unsensitized D-negative woman with D-positive red cells in the course of treating a massive hemorrhage. If the woman is of childbearing age, it is desirable to remove the D-positive red cells, either by giving intravenous anti-D (300 µg per 15 mL of red cells) if the transfusion was limited to 1 to 2 units or by performing an RCE with D-negative product when it becomes available. To minimize the chance of alloimmunization, RCE should be performed as soon as possible after the D-positive transfusions. A two-volume RCE using D-negative blood should reduce the fraction of D-positive cells remaining to about 10% of the starting level.[34] A dose of intravenous Rh Immune Globulin sufficient to prevent alloimmunization caused by the remaining D-positive red cells can then be given. The percentage of circulating cells that are D-positive can be estimated by comparing the reaction with anti-D in the patient's blood to that in a sequence of artificial mixtures of D-positive and -negative cells.[32] Pre- and post-RCE estimates can help plan the size of the exchange and the dose of Rh Immune Globulin, respectively.

RCE has also been used to either prevent or treat hemolysis resulting from ABO-mismatched transfusion, marrow transplantation, or passenger lymphocyte syndrome. Generally, a 1.5 to 2 RCV exchange is performed using compatible red cells.[35]

Intoxication

Carbon Monoxide Poisoning

Carbon monoxide (CO) has a greater affinity for hemoglobin than oxygen does, and, once bound as COHb, it shifts the oxygen dissociation curve to the left, resulting in tissue hypoxemia. CO also binds to myoglobin, certain important cytochrome enzymes, and brain lipids.[36] The half life of COHb is about 320 minutes but decreases with 100% normobaric oxygen therapy. Hyperbaric oxy-

129

gen therapy can further shorten half life; however, it is not readily available.[37] Emergent two-volume RCE along with standard 100% normobaric oxygen therapy may hasten recovery from severe CO intoxication.

Methemoglobinemia

Exchange transfusion has traditionally been recommended for treatment of patients whose acquired methemoglobinemia is refractory to methylene blue. A 1.5 to 2 RCV RCE may successfully diminish the methemoglobin level.[38]

References

1. Pepkowitz S. Red cell exchange and other therapeutic alterations of red cell mass. In: McLeod BC, Price TH, Weinstein R, eds. Apheresis: Principles and practice. 2nd ed. Bethesda, MD: AABB Press, 2003:411-35.
2. Vichinsky EP, Luban NL, Wright E, et al. Prospective RBC phenotype matching in a stroke-prevention trial in sickle cell anemia: A multicenter transfusion trial. Transfusion 2001;41:1086-92.
3. Myers L, Paranjape G, Anderson C, et al. Isovolemic hemodilution-red blood cell exchange (IHD-RBCX) is superior to red blood cell exchange (RBCX) in the management of sickle cell disease (SCD) patients on hypertransfusion programs following cerebrovascular accident (abstract). Blood 2003;102(Suppl):764a.
4. Danielson CF. The role of red blood cell exchange transfusion in the treatment and prevention of complications of sickle cell disease. Ther Apher 2002;6:24-31.
5. Beutler E. The sickle cell diseases and related disorders. In: Beutler E, Lichtman M, Coller B, et al, eds. Williams hematology. 6th ed. New York: McGraw-Hill, 2001:581-605.

6. Hartwig D, Schlager F, Bucsky P, et al. Successful long-term erythrocytapheresis therapy in a patient with symptomatic sickle-cell disease using an arterio-venous fistula. Transfus Med 2002;12:75-7.

7. Smith JW, Weinstein R, Hillyer KL, for the AABB Hemapheresis Committee. Therapeutic apheresis: A summary of current indication categories endorsed by the AABB and the American Society for Apheresis. Transfusion 2003;43: 820-2.

8. McLeod BC. Introduction to the third special issue: Clinical applications of therapeutic apheresis. J Clin Apheresis 2000;15:1-5.

9. Wierenga KJ, Hambleton IR, Lewis NA. Survival estimates for patients with homozygous sickle-cell disease in Jamaica: A clinic-based population study. Lancet 2001; 357:680-3.

10. Ohene-Frempong K, Weiner SJ, Sleeper LA, et al. Cerebrovascular accidents in sickle cell disease: Rates and risk factors. Blood 1998;91:288-94.

11. Ohene-Frempong K. Stroke in sickle cell disease: Demographic, clinical, and therapeutic considerations. Semin Hematol 1991;28:213-9.

12. Kirkham FJ, DeBaun MR. Stroke in children with sickle cell disease. Curr Treat Options Neurol 2004;6:357-75.

13. Kaul DK, Nagel RL, Chen D, Tsai HM. Sickle erythrocyte-endothelial interactions in microcirculation: The role of von Willebrand factor and implications for vasoocclusion. Blood 1993;81:2429-38.

14. Balkaran B, Char G, Morris JS, et al. Stroke in a cohort of patients with homozygous sickle cell disease. J Pediatr 1992;120:360-6.

15. Adams RJ, McKie VC, Hsu L, et al. Prevention of a first stroke by transfusions in children with sickle cell anemia and abnormal results on transcranial Doppler ultrasonography. N Engl J Med 1998;339:5-11.

16. Clinical alert from the National Heart, Lung, and Blood Institute. [Available at http://www.nhlbi.nih.gov/health/proj/blood/sickle/clinical-alert-scd.htm or .pdf.]

131

17. Nietert PJ, Abboud MR, Silverstein MD, Jackson SM. Bone marrow transplantation versus periodic prophylactic blood transfusion in sickle cell patients at high risk of ischemic stroke: A decision analysis. Blood 2000;95: 3057-64.

18. Vichinsky EP, Styles LA, Colangelo LH, et al. Acute chest syndrome in sickle cell disease: Clinical presentation and course. Cooperative Study of Sickle Cell Disease. Blood 1997;89:1787-92.

19. Powars D, Weidman JA, Odom-Maryon T, et al. Sickle cell chronic lung disease: Prior morbidity and the risk of pulmonary failure. Medicine (Baltimore) 1988;67:66-76.

20. Telen MJ. Principles and problems of transfusion in sickle cell disease. Semin Hematol 2001;38:315-23.

21. Davies SC, Olatunji PO. Blood transfusion in sickle cell disease. Vox Sang 1995;68:145-51.

22. Hamre MR, Harmon EP, Kirpatrick DV, et al. Priapism as a complication of sickle cell disease. J Urol 1991;145:1-5.

23. Chakrabarty A, Upadhyay J, Dhabuwala CB, et al. Priapism associated with sickle cell hemoglobinopathy in children: Long-term effects on potency. J Urol 1996;155: 1419-23.

24. Siegel JF, Rich MA, Brock WA. Association of sickle cell disease, priapism, exchange transfusion and neurological events: ASPEN syndrome. J Urol 1993;150:1480-2.

25. Howard RJ, Tuck SM, Pearson TC. Pregnancy in sickle cell disease in the UK: Results of a multicentre survey of the effect of prophylactic blood transfusion on maternal and fetal outcome. Br J Obstet Gynaecol 1995;102: 947-51.

26. Lee W, Werch J, Rokey R, et al. Physiologic observations of pregnant women undergoing prophylactic erythrocytapheresis for sickle cell disease. Transfusion 1991;31:59-62.

27. Koshy M, Weiner SJ, Miller ST, et al. Surgery and anesthesia in sickle cell disease. Cooperative Study of Sickle Cell Diseases. Blood 1995;86:3676-84.

28. Scott-Conner CEH, Brunson CD. The pathophysiology of the sickle hemoglobinopathies and implications for perioperative management. Am J Surg 1994;168:268-74.

29. Vichinsky EP, Haberkern CM, Neumayr L, et al. A comparison of conservative and aggressive transfusion regimens in the perioperative management of sickle cell disease. The Preoperative Transfusion in Sickle Cell Disease Study Group. N Engl J Med 1995;333:206-13.

30. Shulman G, McQuitty C, Vertrees RA, Conti VR. Acute normovolemic red cell exchange for cardiopulmonary bypass in sickle cell disease. Ann Thorac Surg 1998;65: 1444-6.

31. Berdoukas VA, Kwan YL, Sansotta ML. A study on the value of red cell exchange transfusion in transfusion dependent anaemias. Clin Lab Haematol 1986;8:209-20.

32. Zhang Y, Telleria L, Vinetz JM, et al. Erythrocytapheresis for *Plasmodium falciparum* infection complicated by cerebral malaria and hyperparasitemia. J Clin Apheresis 2001; 16:15-8.

33. Machtinger L, Telford SR 3rd, Inducil C, et al. Treatment of babesiosis by red blood cell exchange in an HIV-positive, splenectomized patient. J Clin Apheresis 1993;8: 78-81.

34. Nester TA, Rumsey DM, Howell CC, et al. Prevention of immunization to D+ red blood cells with red blood cell exchange and intravenous Rh immune globulin. Transfusion 2004;44:1720-3.

35. Blacklock HA, Gilmore MJ, Prentice HG, et al. ABO-incompatible bone-marrow transplantation: Removal of red blood cells from donor marrow avoiding recipient antibody depletion. Lancet 1982;ii:1061-4.

36. Weaver LK. Carbon monoxide poisoning. Crit Care Clin 1999;15:297-317.

37. Vreman HJ, Mahoney JJ, Stevenson DK. Carbon monoxide and carboxyhemoglobin. Adv Pediatr 1995;42:303-34.

38. Golden PJ, Weinstein R. Treatment of high-risk, refractory acquired methemoglobinemia with automated red blood cell exchange. J Clin Apheresis 1998;13:28-31.

133

PEDIATRIC THERAPEUTIC APHERESIS

Introduction

Therapeutic apheresis has been used to treat many of the same diseases that affect children as well as adults, and the guidance provided by the American Society for Apheresis (ASFA) and AABB regarding the clinical indications for therapeutic apheresis is also followed for pediatric patients.[1-4] However, available data are often derived from the clinical experience in adults, and extrapolating the conclusions assumes that the clinical course of a disease and therapeutic response to apheresis will not differ in pediatric patients. Moreover, therapeutic apheresis is often adjunctive therapy for critical illnesses with potentially catastrophic consequences, and few controlled trials have been performed to evaluate treatment efficacy in these settings in general or among sick children in particular. There is also a lack of universally accepted treatment schedules and clinical endpoints for therapeutic apheresis procedures, especially for pediatric applications. Consequently, considerable variability in practice exists among the growing number of institutions providing apheresis services for children.

The most common indication for red cell exchange in the pediatric population is sickle cell disease. Therapeutic leukapheresis may be performed to alleviate complications of hyperleukocytosis in children with leukemia in blast crisis. A relatively new application of plasmapheresis is for the treatment of pediatric autoimmune neurologic disorders associated with streptococcal infections. Although the basic principles of therapeutic apheresis for these conditions are the same regardless of the age of the patient, the procedures used for adults must be modified to safely treat young children.[3,4] Special challenges include securing adequate vascular access, maintaining intravascular fluid balance and red cell mass, and recognizing adverse reactions among young patients who may not be able to report their symptoms.

Technical Considerations

Vascular Access

Adequate vascular access is essential to maintain the rate of blood flow required for apheresis procedures. Typically, an 18-gauge or larger caliber needle is needed for the draw line, and a 22-gauge intravenous catheter is needed for the return line. For adults and some adolescents, peripheral veins in the antecubital fossae can be used for single procedures, such as a red cell exchange. Peripheral access is not an option, however, for young children and infants whose veins cannot accommodate the catheters or collapse under the pressure of the blood draw. Central venous access is required for these patients and may be preferable to peripheral access for some adolescents, depending on the urgency of the clinical situation and expected course of treatment. A femoral venous catheter may be placed for a single procedure, for very limited short-term use, or as a temporary measure until another central venous catheter is available. However, their use is associated with a relatively high risk of catheter-related complications. Children requiring multiple or sequential apheresis procedures usually require a temporary percutaneous central line or a surgically implanted, tunneled, central venous catheter to allow for a longer course of treatment.

The catheter must be rigid enough to withstand the negative pressure required to draw blood into the apheresis machine, and the catheter size should be selected according to the size of the patient (Table 12).[3,4] Hemodialysis catheters such as the MedComp catheter (MedComp, Harleysville, PA) are frequently

Table 12. Pediatric Guidelines for Central Venous Catheter Size*

Patient Weight (kg)	Catheter Size (Fr)[†]
<10	7
10-20	8
20-50	9
>50	9 or 11.5

*Modified from Eder and Kim.[3]
[†]For catheter manufactured by MedComp, Harleysville, PA. Sizes may vary for other manufacturers' products.

used in pediatric practice because of their large bore, double lumen, and ability to support the requisite blood flow rates during apheresis procedures. Although Hickman (CR Bard, Murray Hill, NJ), Infuse-a-Port (Uromed, Yverdon-les-Bains, Switzerland), or peripherally inserted central venous catheters (PICC lines) can be used for returning replacement fluids during apheresis procedures, these types of catheters cannot be used to draw blood from a patient into the apheresis machine. Intravascular catheters may be associated with complications including vessel damage, bleeding, infection, or thrombosis. The risks associated with line placement and maintenance should be weighed against the expected benefit of therapeutic apheresis.

Anticoagulation

The approach to anticoagulation may be different for pediatric patients than for adults, depending upon the procedure.[1-4] Citrate is the universally preferred anticoagulant for adults, and is generally well tolerated in children, but alternative regimens utilizing heparin alone or heparin in combination with citrate have been advocated for pediatric use. Citrate is generally preferable to heparin, because it is more rapidly metabolized and does not result in sys-

137

temic anticoagulation. Citrate anticoagulation during plasma-pheresis and red cell exchange is generally well tolerated in children when proper attention is given to the rate of citrate infusion and calcium supplementation.[3-5]

Leukapheresis procedures to collect hematopoietic progenitor cells are particularly associated with citrate toxicity because of the high anticoagulant flow rate and large volume of blood processed; heparin has been recommended as an alternative or adjunct anticoagulant in this setting. However, full-dose citrate anticoagulation with prophylactic intravenous divalent cation infusion was shown to be effective and safe for children undergoing large-volume leukapheresis procedures.[5] Alternatively, a combination of citrate and heparin allows for lower doses of citrate and reduces the risk of citrate toxicity during leukapheresis procedures. Baseline anticoagulation with citrate (1:25 to 1:30 ratio of citrate to whole blood) can be combined with heparin boluses at the beginning of the procedure (20-40 IU/kg) and as needed (10-20 IU/kg) to double the activated clotting time (ACT) from the normal value of 90 seconds to the therapeutic value of 180 seconds.[6] An alternative approach is the continuous administration of heparin during the procedure, by adding heparin directly to an acid-citrate-dextrose (ACD) anticoagulant (10 U heparin/mL ACD) and infusing with low-dose citrate (whole blood-to-anticoagulant ratio of 1:30) without monitoring ACT.[4]

Intravascular Volume and Red Cell Balance

Continuous-flow apheresis devices such as the Spectra (Gambro BCT, Lakewood, CO) are preferred over intermittent-flow devices for pediatric use because of their smaller extracorporeal volumes. The patient's total blood volume (TBV), plasma volume, and/or red cell volume should be calculated before the procedure.[3,4] A weight-based calculation of total blood volume is an acceptable approximation for most patients (Table 13) but may not be an accurate prediction in certain circumstances. For example, the TBV of sick, preterm infants was directly measured by the fetal hemoglobin dilution method and demonstrated wide variability (53-105 mL/kg), suggesting that indirect assessment based on weight may not be accurate.[7] In addition, weight-based estimates may give a

Table 13. Total Blood Volume

Age Group	Approximate Blood Volume (mL/kg)
Premature infant, at birth	90-105
Term newborn infant	80-90
Children (>3 months)	70-75
Adolescents and adults	
Male	70
Female	65

value that is too high for the TBV of extremely obese individuals and a value that is too low for the TBV of lean or muscular individuals.

Automated apheresis devices use more complex algorithms to calculate TBV based on gender, height, and weight. However, this method also has limitations, and the calculation performed by the Spectra (Gambro) was shown to be inaccurate for boys aged 10 to 12 years and weighing less than 30 kg.[8] The TBV calculated automatically for this group of patients should be checked against a weight-based calculation, and the setting on the apheresis machine should be manually adjusted, if necessary.

The calculated TBV is used to evaluate the patient's ability to tolerate the intravascular shifts of fluid and red cells that occur during therapeutic apheresis. At the beginning of a standard procedure, blood is drawn from the patient into the extracorporeal circuit, and the saline contained in the tubing and centrifuge channel is diverted to a waste bag. The blood remaining in the tubing at the end of the procedure is given back to the patient in the "rinseback" phase. The net result is an intravascular volume and red cell deficit during the procedure, followed by the return of most of the red cells along with a net fluid gain at the end. The expected intravascular volume and red cell shifts vary, depending on the device and procedure (Table 14). These volume shifts are usually inconsequential for an adult, but account for proportionately more of a smaller patient's TBV and may not be well tolerated by a young child. In general, the therapeutic goal should be to limit acute intravascular volume changes to no more than 10% to 15% of the patient's TBV.

For example, a 4-year-old girl weighing 15 kg (25th percentile for age) has a total blood volume of 1050 mL (15 kg × 70 mL/kg). If the standard plasmapheresis procedure (eg, Spectra, dual-needle operation) was performed, the prime saline in the extracorporeal circuit would be diverted to the waste bag, and the full rinseback volume would be given at the end of the procedure. The child would experience the following intravascular volume shifts:

$$\text{Intraprocedure volume loss} =$$
$$\text{Value from Table 14} \div \text{TBV} = 150 \text{ mL} \div 1050 \text{ mL} =$$
$$\mathbf{-15\%} \text{ TBV}$$

$$\text{Postprocedure volume gain} =$$
$$\text{Value from Table 14} \div \text{TBV} =$$
$$195 \text{ mL} \div 1050 \text{ mL} = \mathbf{+19\%} \text{ TBV}$$

In this case, the initial loss of 15% of the TBV may not be tolerated, especially in the presence of confounding factors such as dehydration or cardiac, renal, or hepatic dysfunction. Similarly, performing a full rinseback as part of the standard procedure may be problematic, because it will result in a positive fluid balance of an additional 19% TBV at the end of the procedure. The procedure must be adjusted for this patient, to avoid possible untoward effects of these unacceptable intravascular volume shifts. In order to maintain intravascular fluid volume constant as blood is being drawn into the machine, the prime saline should be returned to the patient instead of being diverted to the waste bag, or other replacement fluids should be administered to the patient at the beginning of the procedure. In addition, the rinseback phase

Table 14. Intravascular Volume and Red Cell Shifts*[†]

| | Net Intravascular Volume Shift (mL) | | Net Red Cell Volume Shift (mL)[‡] | |
	Intraprocedure	Postprocedure	Intraprocedure	Postprocedure
Plasmapheresis	−150	+195	−68	−15
Red cell exchange	−100	+245	−68	−16
Leukapheresis, version 4.7	−150 + AC −white cells	+263 + AC − white cells	−114 − [red cell content in collected white cells]	−24 − [red cell content in collected white cells]
Leukapheresis, version 6.0	−150 + AC −white cells	+185 + AC − white cells	−66 − [red cell content in white cells][§]	−9 − [red cell content in white cells][‡]

*Modified from Eder and Kim.[3]

[†]Using the Spectra (Gambro) dual-needle operation, standard procedure (divert saline prime, perform rinseback).

[‡]Volume of blood warmer or other device added to the extracorporeal circuit is not included.

[§]Average red cell content (volume) in white cells collected = volume of white cells collected × hematocrit of white cell product/100.

AC = anticoagulant volume.

141

can be eliminated if a red cell prime was used at the beginning of the procedure.

In general, red cell priming is recommended 1) when drawing whole blood into the extracorporeal circuit will result in depletion of greater than 30% of the patient's original circulating red cell volume or 2) when any degree of reduction in the patient's circulating red cell volume or any impairment of oxygen-carrying capacity is undesirable because of concomitant illness.[3,4] Children weighing less than 20 kg or under 6 years of age usually require red cell priming before apheresis, as do older children with anemia or underlying cardiopulmonary disease, hemodynamic instability, or tissue ischemia. The amount of donor blood needed to maintain the patient's hematocrit at an acceptable level during the procedure should be calculated.

For example, a 4-year-old child weighing 15 kg with a baseline hematocrit of 30% and a 1050-mL TBV will require a red cell prime for a modified plasmapheresis procedure (eg, Spectra, dual-needle operation) as shown in Table 15.

Priming just the return line with the required volume of red cells is preferred to priming the entire extracorporeal circuit with a Red Blood Cell (RBC) unit, because it uses less donor blood and provides better control over the volume of red cells delivered to the patient. If less than a full donor RBC unit is needed for a procedure, a sterile connection device should be used to prepare the aliquot so that the remaining portion of the unit can be reserved for the same patient. The red cell prime can be prepared as an unmanipulated aliquot from a donor RBC unit [hematocrit 55-65% for unit of AS (Additive Solution) RBCs], which will transiently raise the patient's hematocrit at the beginning of the procedure, or by reconstituting the donor red cells with a diluent to the same hematocrit as the patient, which will maintain a constant hematocrit throughout the procedure. The choice of diluent depends on the clinical situation, but the options include 0.9% NaCl, 5% albumin, or Fresh Frozen Plasma (FFP) if clotting factors are also needed by the patient. The use of a reconstituted prime is not often clinically necessary but may be indicated for a therapeutic leukapheresis procedure to treat symptomatic hyperleukocytosis. It avoids raising the patient's hematocrit and fur-

Table 15. Sample Calculations for Red Cell Priming*

Red Cell Parameter	Formula and Calculation	
Total red cell volume	TBV × hematocrit = 1050 mL (0.30) = 315 mL	
Intraprocedure red cell loss (Volume of extracorporeal circuit × hematocrit of blood in circuit)	From Table 14 Blood warmer (SpectraTherm) Total red cell loss =	68 mL + 36 mL 104 mL
Predicted hematocrit of patient during isovolemic procedure (ie, return prime saline)	(315 mL − 104 mL) ÷ 1050 = 20%	
Volume of donor red cells needed to maintain patient hematocrit at 30% during procedure (donor red cell unit, 55% hematocrit)	104 ÷ (0.55) = 189 mL	

*For a 4-year-old child weighing 15 kg with a baseline hematocrit of 30% and a total blood volume (TBV) of 1050 mL.

ther increasing the viscosity of the patient's blood, which could aggravate symptoms of leukostasis.

To prepare reconstituted blood to prime the return line in the example given in Table 15, the volume of diluent needed should be calculated as follows:

$$\text{Volume of donor red cells needed}$$
$$\text{(at 55\% hematocrit)} = 189 \text{ mL}$$

$$\text{Final total volume} = 189 \text{ mL} \times 0.55 \div 0.3 = 347 \text{ mL}$$

$$\text{Volume of diluent needed} =$$
$$\text{Final total volume} - \text{starting volume} =$$
$$347 \text{ mL} - 189 \text{ mL} = 158 \text{ mL}$$

If a red cell prime is given at the beginning of the procedure, the final rinseback phase is often omitted to avoid volume overload. Alternatively, a partial rinseback volume of up to 15% of the patient's TBV may be given, if the therapeutic goal is to further increase the patient's hematocrit and if the patient can tolerate the additional volume. For example, giving 150 mL of the rinseback (hematocrit, 30%) in the 15-kg patient will provide the equivalent of 81 mL of a donor RBC unit (hematocrit, 55%) or about 5 mL/kg, which would be expected to increase the patient's hematocrit by about 3 percentage points (or increase hemoglobin by about 1 g/dL). If partial rinseback is given, or if a reconstituted red cell prime is used, the additional volume administered to the patient must be factored into the equation to calculate the intravascular fluid balance during the procedure. Similarly, infusions of other medications during the procedure must also be taken into consideration when accounting for intravascular volume balance.

Adverse Reactions

Adverse reactions during therapeutic apheresis procedures may be related to the anticoagulant, volume shifts, transfused blood components, or anxiety and must be promptly recognized and appropriately treated.

Children may be more anxious about therapeutic apheresis than adults. This tendency must be anticipated and handled in a manner consistent with the developmental stage of the child. Distraction techniques (such as videos, games, or simple play) are useful to divert the child's attention away from the procedure and minimize anxiety.

Citrate-induced hypocalcemia is often manifest as perioral tingling or numbness and paresthesias in adults; however, children rarely report these symptoms. More commonly, children experience nausea and vomiting as the first indication of citrate toxicity. Blood pressure changes may also signal citrate toxicity, and vital signs should be carefully monitored during pediatric procedures, especially for children who are unable to articulate their symptoms. Severe hypocalcemia may be associated with frank tetany, electrocardiogram abnormalities, and dysrhythmias. Serum concentrations of ionized calcium should be measured during suspected reactions or before the procedure in patients at risk for hypocalcemia. Symptoms of hypocalcemia can be treated by slowing the rate of citrate infusion, pausing the procedure, and/or administering calcium. Oral calcium may be given, but its efficacy in treating citrate reactions has not been demonstrated. Intravenous calcium supplementation is necessary for immediate correction of serum ionized calcium in treatment of severe citrate reactions. Apheresis instruments have preprogrammed limits on the anticoagulant flow rate and minimum volume that can be safely processed. These parameters can be manually overridden, but doing so requires careful consideration of procedural adjustments needed to minimize citrate toxicity in small patients, as well as consideration of the amount of blood that will be needed to prime the extracorporeal circuit relative to the patient's TBV. Calcium supplementation is generally required if the anticoagulant flow rate is greater than 0.8 mL/minute during any apheresis procedure. Because of the limitations of the equipment, manual exchange transfusion is often preferable to automated exchange procedures for children less than 1 year old.

Vasovagal reactions present with pallor, diaphoresis, and hypotension. Hypotension may otherwise be caused by hypovolemia, but the two reactions can be distinguished by the pulse rate: bradycardia occurs in vasovagal reactions; tachycardia, with hypovolemia. Vasovagal reactions are treated by pausing the procedure and placing the patient in the Trendelenberg position (ie, supine with head lower than legs). Hypovolemic reactions are also treated with administration of additional replacement fluids or a saline bolus. A dilutional coagulopathy may develop following multiple closely spaced or sequential plasma exchange procedures using colloid or crystalloid for fluid replacement. Clinical and laboratory evaluation before the procedure should determine if plasma components should be included as the final replacement fluid during the procedure.

Red Cell Exchange

Sickle Cell Disease

Sickle cell disease is characterized by acute and chronic complications of anemia, vascular occlusion, and thrombosis. The role of red cell transfusion is widely accepted for treating severe crises, such as stroke and acute chest syndrome, and preventing chronic complications, although the therapeutic goals can been achieved with either red cell exchange or simple transfusion.[9]

The goals of red cell transfusion in treating acute complications of sickle cell disease are to reduce or prevent sickling by lowering HbS concentration and to increase oxygen delivery to tissues by increasing the hematocrit. The choice of red cell exchange or simple transfusion for a given indication varies from center to center. In a recent study involving 538 sickle cell patients treated for acute chest syndrome at 30 centers, the majority of transfused patients received simple transfusions compared to only about a third who received exchange transfusion.[10] Both methods resulted in statistically significant improvements in oxygenation. Nevertheless, red cell exchange offers theoretical advantages over simple transfusion in the setting of treatment of acute thrombotic complications. Simple transfusion increases blood viscosity, which may increase the risk of further vascular occlusion in previously untransfused patients or those with predominantly HbS. Red cell exchange increases hematocrit while removing HbS and avoids the risk of unfavorable effect on the circulation. In addition, sickle cell patients with compensated anemia may develop circulatory overload and cardiac compromise with the volume expansion associated with simple transfusion, and patients with coexistent cardiac disease or renal compromise are at greatest risk. Red cell exchange avoids volume overload because the patient's fluid balance can be controlled during the procedure to closely approximate euvolemic conditions.

If red cell exchange is performed to treat severe complications of sickle cell disease, the patient's HbS should be reduced to less than 30% of the total hemoglobin, and the hematocrit at the end of the procedure should be increased to about 30%. Hematocrits greater than 36% in children with sickle cell disease have been linked to serious thrombotic complications, likely the result of altered rheological properties of whole blood. If the patient has not been transfused within the previous 3 months, the pre-exchange HbS level can be assumed to be 100%. Exchange of one blood volume should raise the HbA level to about 65% and lower HbS to about 35%; consequently, slightly more than one red cell volume should be exchanged so that the fraction of cells remaining (FCR) is less than 30%. The apheresis instrument calculates the volume of donor red cells needed for the procedure based on the patient's TBV and desired FCR, but an initial manual estimate is often required in advance to alert the blood bank to the approximate number of units that will be needed for the procedure. For example, a 9-year-old, 29-kg child with a blood volume of 2030 mL, a hematocrit of 25%, and a red cell volume of 508 mL (29 kg × 70 mL/kg) will require approximately 3 units of AS-RBCs (Average donor unit red cell content = unit hematocrit (55%) × unit volume (330 mL) = 0.55 × 330 mL = 180 mL red cells/unit; number of units needed = patient red cell volume ÷ unit red cell content = 508 mL ÷ 180 mL/unit = 3 units). Postexchange hematocrit and hemoglobin electrophoresis should be performed to validate the efficiency of the exchange.

Chronic transfusion therapy to maintain the patient's HbS level between 30% and 50% of the total hemoglobin is recommended not only to prevent recurrent stroke, but also to prevent the first occurrence of stroke in patients at risk as determined by abnormal results on transcranial Doppler ultrasonography.[11,12] Although the therapeutic goal can be achieved with a regular schedule of simple transfusion, iron overload is an inevitable consequence that necessitates chelation therapy with daily infusions of desferoximine, a therapy with which many patients are noncompliant. If not treated, iron overload will impair cardiac function, cause endocrine disturbance, and lead to multiorgan failure. In contrast, red cell exchange reduces iron accumulation compared to simple transfusion and obviates the need for iron chelation therapy in some chronically transfused patients.[13-16]

For pediatric stroke patients, the aim in the first 3 years of chronic transfusion therapy is to maintain HbS below 30% of the total hemoglobin.[3,4] If a patient is stable on this regimen for 3 years, the treatment goal may be relaxed to maintain HbS less than 50% of the total hemoglobin to achieve comparable clinical benefit. Partial red cell exchange to replace 40% to 60% of a patient's red cell mass can be performed every 3 to 4 weeks when the HbS goal is less than 30% or every 4 to 5 weeks when the HbS goal is less than 50%. Isovolemic hemodilution (see more detail in the section on Red Cell Exchange) may be performed safely at the beginning of the procedure, to remove the patient's sickled cells. Saline is infused as the sickled cells are removed before starting the red cell exchange with donor units. This reduces the amount of donor blood needed to achieve the desired reduction in HbS.[17] Isovolemic hemodilution should be used only if the patient is on a chronic treatment schedule and is otherwise healthy; it should not be used in the setting of acute stroke or other emergencies. The target hematocrit following red cell exchange is either 27% or the same as the patient's preprocedure hematocrit but less than 36%, to prevent hyperviscosity and to optimize iron balance. Chronic transfusion therapy to prevent stroke is a likely a lifetime commitment, because the risk returns to baseline when long-term transfusion therapy is discontinued.[12] At many centers in the United States, exchange transfusion is preferred because the benefit of preventing stroke and iron-induced organ damage outweighs the risks associated with exchange transfusion.

Red cell exchange transfusion requires more donor blood than simple transfusion to achieve the same fractional reduction in HbS in chronically transfused patients. Increased donor exposure is accompanied by greater risk of virus transmission, red cell alloimmunization, and delayed hemolytic transfusion reactions. Delayed hemolytic transfusion reactions, usually mild in most clinical settings, may result in severe life-threatening anemia in patients with sickle cell disease.[18] The risk of alloimmunization is reduced by providing units that are matched to the patient with respect to blood group antigen expression in the Rh, Kell, and other systems. By prospectively matching for C, E, and K1 blood group antigens, the alloimmunization rate among chronically transfused sickle cell patients was reduced from 3% to 0.5% per unit, and hemolytic transfusion reactions were reduced by 90%.[19] This strategy is becoming more widely accepted, but an alternative approach restricts the use of phenotypically matched red cells to patients who have become immunized to one red cell antigen and are at risk of developing additional alloantibodies and autoantibodies.[18]

RBC units intended for sickle cell patients should be screened for sickle trait, and HbS-negative units should be selected for transfusion. This simplifies evaluation of the percentage of HbS in the patient's circulation after exchange transfusion. In addition, it avoids the potential risk that red cells from a blood donor with sickle trait may not function normally under conditions of hypoxia, acidosis, and dehydration present in critically ill patients in an acute sickle crisis. Leukocyte reduction of cellular components is indicated for sickle cell transfusion recipients, primarily for prevention of recurrent febrile nonhemolytic transfusion reactions. Gamma irradiation of units selected for transfusion to sickle cell patients is not required, unless there is a coexistent medical condition, such as marrow transplantation, that places them at risk of transfusion-associated graft-vs-host disease.

AABB and ASFA classify red cell exchange as a Category I indication for sickle cell disease, although indications for specific applications of red cell exchange in treating or preventing the various complications of sickle cell disease have not yet been described.[1,2]

Therapeutic Apheresis for Red Cell Removal

Automated erythrocytapheresis may be performed as an alternative to manual phlebotomy in specific clinical situations. Red cell removal is generally indicated to alleviate symptoms attributable to increased red cell mass in polycythemia vera or secondary polycythemia resulting from cyanotic congenital heart disease and to reduce iron stores in hemochromatosis.[20] During erythrocytapheresis, the patient's red cells can be removed and simultaneously replaced with a plasma substitute such as 5% albumin to maintain constant intravascular volume during the procedure.

While simple phlebotomy is more often performed for these indications, a continuous isovolemic procedure may be better tolerated than discontinuous manual phlebotomy by hemodynamically unstable children or those with significant cardiac disease. AABB and ASFA classify phlebotomy as a Category I indication and erythrocytapheresis as a Category II indication for erythrocytosis/polycythemia vera.[1,2]

Plasmapheresis

Plasmapheresis efficiently reduces the plasma concentration of pathogenic antibodies, immune complexes, plasma proteins, cytokines, lipoproteins, protein-bound drugs, or metabolic toxins.[20,21] Consequently, plasmapheresis has been used to treat a wide variety of diseases in both children and adults. Indications that occur in both children and adults but are more likely to affect adults are covered in the section on Therapeutic Plasma Exchange. Diseases that present in the pediatric age group in which plasmapheresis has a unique role include pediatric autoimmune neuropsychiatric disorders associated with streptococcal infections (PANDAS), atypical hemolytic uremic syndrome (HUS), thrombotic thrombocytopenic purpura (TTP), Rasmussen's encephalitis, familial hypercholesterolemia, and phytanic acid storage disease (Refsum's disease).

Pediatric Autoimmune Neurologic Disorders Associated with Streptococcal Infections

PANDAS is a relatively new indication for plasmapheresis. Affected children have tics and obsessive-compulsive disorder (OCD), and they experience behavioral exacerbations following infection with group A beta-hemolytic streptococcus (GABHS).[22] Antibodies directed against GABHS are postulated to cross-react with neuronal cells to produce inflammation in the central nervous system (CNS), particularly within the basal ganglia, in patients with PANDAS. Perlmutter et al randomly assigned 30 children with severe PANDAS to receive either plasma exchange, intravenous immune globulin (IVIG), or placebo (saline infusion).[23] The plasma exchange group received five single-volume exchanges over 2 weeks, with 5% albumin and saline replacement. Plasma exchange and IVIG were both effective in lessening the severity of symptoms in affected children. Symptomatic improvement persisted for most children in both active treatment groups for at least 1 year, with a trend toward greater relief of OCD symptoms with plasma exchange than with IVIG.

AABB and ASFA classify PANDAS as a Category II indication for plasma exchange.

Atypical TTP/HUS

Classic HUS is characterized by the acute onset of thrombocytopenia, microangiopathic hemolytic anemia, and renal dysfunction, and it accounts for approximately 90% of childhood HUS cases. Symptoms usually develop following a diarrheal illness, most often caused by enterotoxigenic bacteria, such as *Escherichia coli* O157:H7. The vast majority of children with classic HUS recover fully with supportive treatment and dialysis, do not require plasmapheresis, and do not experience relapses or recurrences.

The remaining 10% of cases of childhood HUS are referred to variously as atypical, non-diarrhea-associated, or sporadic HUS. A proportion of these cases are likely caused by invasive pneumococcal infection; other cases are idiopathic or secondary to drugs, malignancy, marrow transplantation, or systemic infections.[24-27] Pneumococcal-associated HUS is treated with supportive care and dialysis, and some authors caution against transfusing plasma-containing blood components to these patients.[24,25] Clinically, atypical HUS in children resembles TTP in adults, in that neurologic features may dominate the clinical picture. Because of the difficulty in distinguishing HUS and TTP and the extremely poor prognosis if left untreated, prompt initiation of plasma exchange is recommended for atypical HUS or for patients with thrombotic microangiopathic hemolytic anemia if there is doubt about the cause.[27,28] In TTP, plasma exchange effectively removes offending inhibitors of von Willebrand factor (vWF) metalloprotease activity (ADAMTS13) if these are present and replenishes functional enzyme which cleaves unusually large vWF and renders it less thrombogenic.[28-30] The mechanism of benefit, if any, in HUS is unknown.

Treatment for atypical TTP/HUS requires daily plasma exchange and replacement of 1 to 1.5 plasma volumes with FFP or Plasma Cryoprecipitate Reduced (ie, cryosupernatant, cryopoor plasma), ideally until the patient's lactate dehydrogenase normalizes and the platelet count increases to greater than $100,000/\mu L$ for 2 to 3 consecutive days.[28,31] The duration of treatment necessary to effect a response among adults with TTP is variable, but it averages 10 days with a range of 2 to 34 days.[31] If a patient experiences an acute exacerbation of TTP following withdrawal of treatment or a recurrence of the disease several weeks after treatment, plasmapheresis must be emergently resumed.

AABB and ASFA classify TTP as a Category I indication for plasma exchange; in contrast, HUS is a Category III indication for plasma exchange, which primarily reflects the heterogenous pediatric and adult patient populations that have been described to date.[1,2]

Chronic relapsing TTP in children is a rare disease caused by a congenital deficiency of ADAMTS13.[32] Enzyme replacement with regular infusions of plasma is adequate treatment, and plasmapheresis is not required.

Rasmussen's Encephalitis

Rasmussen's encephalitis is a rare, progressive neurologic disorder that occurs in children under 10 years of age.[33] Affected children have frequent and severe seizures that are localized to one cerebral hemisphere, leading to the loss of motor skills and speech and ultimately to hemiparesis, mental retardation, and dementia. Antiepileptic drugs are not effective at controlling seizures, and intractable epilepsy is accompanied by loss of function in the affected cerebral hemisphere. The etiology of the disease is unknown, but many affected patients have autoantibodies that recognize the Glu R3 receptor for the CNS neurotransmitter glutamate.[34] A possible model is molecular mimicry, which holds that antecedent viral infection results in the production of cross-reactive autoantibodies. The striking localization of neurologic deterioration to a single hemisphere may reflect focal disruption of the blood-brain barrier that permits the pathogenic antibodies to enter the brain and elicit seizure activity.[33] This seizure activity aggravates the damage to the blood-brain barrier and cerebral cortex and propagates a vicious cycle of unrelenting seizures.

Plasmapheresis has been used as an adjunct or alternative to medical treatment (eg, steroids and IVIG) or surgical treatment (eg, hemispherectomy). Plasmapheresis, in combination with steroids and IVIG, reduces seizure frequency and improves neurologic function in some patients.[35] An initial course of five or six plasma exchanges (1.0 plasma volume) over 10 to 12 days using 5% human serum albumin/0.9% NaCl as replacement fluid has been recommended, to be followed by administration of IVIG (1 g/kg) immediately after the final plasma exchange and again the next day.[33,35] This course of treatment may be required every 2 to 3 months, and steroid administration may permit longer intervals between courses.

AABB and ASFA classify Rasmussen's encephalitis as a Category III indication for plasma exchange.[1,2]

Familial Hypercholesterolemia

Children with familial hypercholesterolemia or severely dyslipidemic patients whose diseases are resistant to diet and drug therapy may benefit from regular plasmapheresis to remove offending total cholesterol, low-density lipoprotein (LDL), and other apolipoprotein-B-containing lipoproteins. Although selective adsorption procedures to remove LDL have been used in some children, the devices (eg, Liposorber, Kaneka, Osaka, Japan) have a relatively large extracorporeal volume that limits their use in pediatric practice.[36] Consequently, regular plasmapheresis may be required until a child reaches adolescence and is better able to tolerate the selective adsorption procedures (see section on Selective Depletion).

AABB and ASFA classify familial hypercholesterolemia as a Category II indication for plasma exchange.[1,2]

Phytanic Acid Storage Disease

Phytanic acid storage disease (Refsum's disease) is an autosomal recessive condition characterized by a deficiency in α-oxidase. The enzyme deficiency reduces the ability to metabolize phytanic acid, a dietary lipid. Accumulation of phytanic acid in the body leads to the clinical disorder heredopathia atactica polyneuritiformis, which is characterized by multiple neurologic manifestations including retinitis pigmentosa, peripheral neuropathy, cerebellar ataxia, sensorineural deafness, and anosmia.[21] Additional findings include ichthyosis, skeletal problems, and cardiac arrhythmias. The onset of symptoms is variable and may occur in childhood or adulthood. Elevation in phytanic acid occurs in relation to concurrent illnesses or weight loss, probably due to mobilization from adipose tissue.

Dietary restriction of animal sources of phytanic acid is the cornerstone of therapy. Serum lipoproteins serve as carriers for excessive phytanic acid in patients, and plasmapheresis is a useful adjunct to dietary treatment.[21] Symptomatic improvement has been reported in most patients treated with plasma exchange in case reports; however, cranial nerve involvement and sensory deficits do not respond to treatment. Plasmapheresis has been used to treat acute and life-threatening complications of phytanic acid storage disease, such as arrythmias and conduction disturbances, which respond quickly to reduction of serum phytanic acid levels. There are no controlled trials on the use of plasma exchange in the treatment of phytanic acid storage disease, but the generally accepted approach involves one or two single-volume plasma exchanges per week for 3 to 6 weeks or until symptomatic improvement, using 5% albumin for fluid replacement. Membrane differential filtration apheresis is also effective treatment of acute exacerbations in case reports, largely due to the fact that phytanic acid circulates bound to lipoproteins, which can be selectively removed in the procedures as described in the section on Selective Depletion.

AABB and ASFA classify phytanic acid storage disease as a Category I indication for plasma exchange or membrane differential filtration apheresis.[1,2]

Leukapheresis

Therapeutic leukapheresis is performed to remove white cells from children with leukemia who have extreme peripheral leukocytosis, often with white cell counts in excess of 100,000/µL, and attendant thrombotic and hemorrhagic complications. Symptoms of hyperleukocytosis reflect impaired blood flow through pulmonary and cerebral vasculature and include tachypnea, dyspnea, pulmonary insufficiency, blurred vision, diplopia, dizziness, slurred speech, and coma. Intracranial or pulmonary hemorrhage is a dire complication of hyperleukocytosis. The risk of symptomatic leukocytosis is greatest for children with acute myeloid leukemia (AML), followed by the accelerated or blast crisis of chronic myelogenous leukemia (CML), acute lymphoblastic leukemia (ALL), chronic phase CML (uncommon), and, finally, chronic lymphocytic leukemia (CLL), in which complications from leukostasis are rare.[37,38] Children are more likely than adults to experience hyperleukocytosis and leukostasis in CML.[39]

The decision to initiate leukapheresis must be individualized and should not be based on an arbitrary white cell threshold. Peripheral cell counts may be extraordinarily high in ALL but are seldom accompanied by symptoms of hyperleukocytosis. A lesser degree of leukocytosis in AML may cause pronounced symptoms of leukostasis. As a general guideline, children with peripheral white cell counts greater than 100,000/µL, a high percentage of blasts and promyelocytes, and neurologic or pulmonary manifestations of leukostasis are candidates for leukocyte depletion. Leukapheresis is a temporizing measure, and definitive treatment of the underlying disease should be coordinated soon after the procedure(s) is/are completed.[40]

Daily leukapheresis procedures may be performed until symptoms improve or until the leukocyte count is substantially reduced and definitive treatment with chemotherapy is under way. The procedure goal must also be individualized. The efficacy of the cytoreduction is variable and reflects total-body tumor burden, proliferative rate, and other physical properties of the leukemic cells and the response to concomitant chemotherapy as well as the volume of blood processed (see Cytapheresis section). Calculation of expected volume shifts before the procedure begins is extremely important to avoid hypovolemia, dehydration, and acid-base imbalance, especially in small children.[3,4] These calculations must take into account the volume of anticoagulant administered and the volume of white cells collected (Table 14). The predicted dose of anticoagulant will depend on the volume of blood processed, rate of anticoagulant infusion, ratio of whole blood to anticoagulant, and plan for calcium supplementation. An example of the volume shifts that could occur during a leukapheresis procedure is given in Table 16 for a 9-year-old girl (29 kg; TBV, 2030 mL) newly diagnosed with T-cell ALL, who presented with an altered level of consciousness, a white cell count of 793,000/µL (90% blasts), and a hematocrit of 26%. To process three blood volumes (6090 mL) on the Spectra (Gambro), version 6.0 software, the predicted final volume collected was 1193 mL (hematocrit of collected product, 7%), using 460 mL anticoagulant.

Unlike a standard plasmapheresis procedure, therapeutic leukapheresis procedures will result in a significant net volume and red cell loss. Fluid balance must be carefully planned to compensate for this predicted loss and to maintain isovolemia. Intravenous calcium supplementation is almost invariably required, and this volume of calcium/normal saline administered will be part of the replacement fluid infused. FFP and platelets were used for the balance of the replacement fluid in the above example because of the risk of CNS hemorrhage. In addition, most children with hyperleukocytosis associated with leukemia are also severely anemic. However, red cell transfusion increases blood viscosity, may further impair perfusion and aggravate leukostasis, and should not be given before the leukapheresis procedure unless there is an overriding need to increase oxygen-carrying capacity. In the example in Table 16, the lowest hematocrit observed during the procedure was 20%, which was close to the predicted intraprocedural value, and the patient tolerated the procedure without a red cell prime. If a red cell prime is used, it should be reconstituted to the same hematocrit as the patient, as previously described. A better alternative may be to transfuse red cells after completion of the leukapheresis proce-

Table 16. Sample Calculations for Volume Shifts during Leukapheresis*

Intravascular Volume Shifts	Formula and Calculation
Postprocedure volume loss (Table 14)	185 mL + anticoagulant − white cells
	185 mL + 460 mL − 1193 mL = −548 mL
% Total blood volume	% TBV = −548 mL ÷ 2030 mL = −27%

Red Cell Balance	Formula and Calculation
Total red cell volume	TBV × hematocrit
	2030 mL (0.26) = 528 mL
Intraprocedure red cell loss (maximum)	From Table 14:
	−66 − [red cell content of white cells] = −66 mL − [volume of white cells collected × hematocrit of white cell product/100] = −66 mL − [1193 mL × 0.07] = −150 mL
Predicted intraprocedure hematocrit nadir of patient with isovolemic procedure	[528 mL − 150 mL] ÷ 2030 = 19%
Postprocedure red cell loss (after rinseback)	From Table 14:
	−9−[red cell content of white cells] = −9 mL − [volume of white cells collected × hematocrit of white cell product/100] = −9 mL − [1193 mL × 0.07] = −93 mL
Predicted postprocedure hematocrit of patient with isovolemic procedure	[528 mL − 93 mL] ÷ 2030 = 21%

*For a 9-year-old girl weighing 29 kg with a hematocrit of 26% and a total blood volume (TBV) of 2030 mL (see text for additional details).

dure, if necessary. The final hematocrit for the patient in the example at the end of the procedure was 22%, and the patient was cautiously transfused with 2.5 mL/kg of a donor RBC unit to a final hematocrit of 24%. Clinical and laboratory monitoring of citrate toxicity is important during leukapheresis procedures; blood flow rates may need to be adjusted during the procedure and intravenous calcium supplementation is usually required. As previously mentioned, heparin may be used in combination with citrate to decrease the dose of citrate and the attendant risk of citrate toxicity in children. Contraindications to heparin use in this setting include significant coagulopathy, hemorrhage, or risk of CNS hemorrhage.

AABB and ASFA classify leukocytosis as a Category I indication for leukapheresis.[1,2]

References

1. McLeod BC. Introduction to the third special issue: Clinical applications of therapeutic apheresis. J Clin Apheresis 2000;15:1-5.
2. Smith JW, Weinstein R, Hillyer KL, et al for the AABB Hemapheresis Committee. Therapeutic apheresis: A summary of current indication categories endorsed by the AABB and American Society for Apheresis. Transfusion 2003;43:820-2.
3. Eder AF, Kim HC. Pediatric therapeutic apheresis. In: Herman JH, Manno CS, eds. Pediatric transfusion therapy. Bethesda, MD: AABB Press, 2000:471-508.
4. Kim HC. Therapeutic pediatric apheresis. J Clin Apheresis 2000;15:129-57.
5. Bolan CD, Yau YY, Cullis HC, et al. Pediatric large-volume leukapheresis: A single institution experience with heparin versus citrate-based anticoagulant regimens. Transfusion 2004;44:229-38.
6. Gorlin JB, Humphreys D, Kent P, et al. Pediatric large volume peripheral blood progenitor cell collections from pa-

tients under 25 kg: A primer. J Clin Apheresis 1996;11: 195-203.

7. Aladangady N, Aitchison TC, Beckett C, et al. Is it possible to predict the blood volume of a sick preterm infant? Arch Dis Child Fetal Neonatal Ed 2004;89:F344-7.

8. Clough L, Dugan N, Hulitt C, et al. Improved method to estimate total blood volume for erythrocytapheresis using the Cobe Spectra in pediatric sickle cell patients (abstract). J Clin Apheresis 1998;13:81.

9. National Heart, Lung, and Blood Institute. The management of sickle cell disease. 4th ed. NIH Publication No. 02-2117. Bethesda, MD: National Institutes of Health, 2002.

10. Vichinsky EP, Neumayr LD, Earles AN, et al. Causes and outcomes of the acute chest syndrome in sickle cell disease. N Engl J Med 2000;342:1855-65.

11. Adams RJ, McKie VC, Hsu L, et al. Prevention of a first stroke by transfusions in children with sickle cell anemia and abnormal results on transcranial Doppler ultrasonography. N Engl J Med 1998;339:5-11.

12. Wang WC, Kovnar EH, Tonkin IL, et al. High risk of recurrent stroke after discontinuance of five to twelve years of transfusion therapy in patients with sickle cell disease. J Pediatr 1991;118:377-82.

13. Kim HC, Dugan NP, Silber JH, et al. Erythrocytapheresis therapy to reduce iron overload in chronically transfused patients with sickle cell disease. Blood 1994;83:1136-42.

14. Adams DM, Schultz WH, Ware RE, Kinney TR. Erythrocytapheresis can reduce iron overload and prevent the need for chelation therapy in chronically transfused pediatric patients. J Pediatr Hematol Oncol 1996;18:46-50.

15. Singer ST, Quirolo K, Niski K, et al. Erythrocytapheresis for chronically transfused children with sickle cell disease: An effective method for maintaining a low hemoglobin S level and reducing iron overload. J Clin Apheresis 1999; 14:122-5.

16. Hilliard LM, Williams BF, Lounsbury AE, Howard TH. Erythrocytapheresis limits iron accumulation in chroni-

cally transfused sickle cell patients. Am J Hematol 1998;
59:28-35.

17. Kim HC, Dugan N, Clough L, et al. Comparison of
erythrocytapheresis performed by intermittent-flow
centrifugation (Haemonetics V50) and continuous-flow
centrifugation (Cobe Spectra) (abstract). J Clin Apheresis
1995;10:41.

18. Smith-Whitley K. Alloimmunization in patients with
sickle cell disease. In: Herman JH, Manno CS, eds. Pediatric transfusion therapy. Bethesda, MD: AABB Press,
2002:249-82.

19. Vichinsky EP, Luban NLC, Wright E, et al. Prospective
RBC phenotype matching in a stroke-prevention trial in
sickle cell anemia: A multicenter transfusion trial. Transfusion 2001;41:1086-92.

20. Grima KM. Therapeutic apheresis in hematological and
oncological diseases. J Clin Apheresis 2000;15:28-52.

21. Winters JL, Pineda AA, McLeod BC, Grima KM. Therapeutic apheresis in renal and metabolic diseases. J Clin
Apheresis 2000;15:53-73.

22. Swedo SE, Leonard HL, Garvey M, et al. Pediatric autoimmune neuropsychiatric disorders associated with streptococcal infections: Clinical description of the first 50
cases. Am J Psychiatry 1998:155:264-71.

23. Perlmutter SJ, Leitman SF, Garvey MA, et al. Therapeutic
plasma exchange and intravenous immunoglobulin for obsessive-compulsive disorder and tic disorders in childhood. Lancet 1999;354:1153-8.

24. Cabrera GR, Fortenberry J, Warshaw BL, et al. Hemolytic
uremic syndrome associated with invasive *Streptococcus
pneumoniae* infection. Pediatrics 1998;101:699-703.

25. Crookston KP, Reiner AP, Cooper RA, et al. RBC T activation and hemolysis: Implications for pediatric transfusion management. Transfusion 2000;40:801-12.

26. Schriber JR, Herzig GP. Transplantation-associated
thrombotic thrombocytopenic purpura and hemolytic
uremic syndrome. Semin Hematol 1997;34:126-33.

27. Slavicek J, Puretic Z, Novak M, et al. The role of plasma exchange in the treatment of severe forms of HUS in childhood. Int J Artif Organs 1995;19:506-10.

28. Sadler JE, Moake JL, Miyata T, George JN. Recent advances in thrombotic thrombocytopenic purpura. Hematology (Am Soc Hematol Educ Program) 2004:407-23.

29. Furlan M, Robles R, Galbusera M, et al. Von Willebrand factor-cleaving protease in thrombotic thrombocytopenic purpura and the hemolytic-uremic syndrome. N Engl J Med 1998;339:1578-84.

30. Tsai HM, Lian ECY. Antibodies to von Willebrand factor-cleaving protease in acute thrombotic thrombocytopenic purpura. N Engl J Med 1998;339:1585-94.

31. Bandarenko N, Brecher ME. United States thrombotic thrombocytopenic purpura apheresis study group (US TTP ASG): Multicenter survey and retrospective analysis of current efficacy of therapeutic plasma exchange. J Clin Apheresis 1998;13:133-41.

32. Chintagumpala MM, Hurwitz RL, Moake JL, et al. Chronic relapsing thrombotic thrombocytopenic purpura in infants with large von Willebrand factor multimers during remission. J Pediatr 1992;120:49-53.

33. Weinstein R. Therapeutic apheresis in neurological disorders. J Clin Apheresis 2000;15:28-52.

34. Rodgers SW, Andrews PI, Gahring LC, et al. Autoantibodies to glutamate receptor Glu R3 in Rasmussen's encephalitis. Science 1994;265:648-51.

35. Andrews PI, Dichter MA, Berkovic SF, et al. Plasmapheresis in Rasmussen's encephalitis. Neurology 1996;46:242-6.

36. Zwiener RJ, Uauy R, Petruska ML, Huet BA. Low-density lipoprotein apheresis as long-term treatment for children with homozygous familial hypercholesterolemia. J Pediatr 1995;126:728-35.

37. Lichtman MA, Rowe JM. Hyperleukocytic leukemias: Rheological, clinical and therapeutic considerations. Blood 1982;60:279-83.

38. Bunin NJ, Pui CH. Differing complications of hyper-leukocytosis in children with acute lymphoblastic or acute nonlymphoblastic leukemia. J Clin Oncol 1985; 3:1590-5.

39. Rowe J, Lichtman M. Hyperleukocytosis and leukostasis: Common features of childhood chronic myelogenous leukemia. Blood 1984;63:1230-4.

40. Lane TA. Continuous-flow leukapheresis for rapid cyto-reduction in leukemia. Transfusion 1980;20:455-7.

SELECTIVE DEPLETION

Introduction

The bulk replacement of plasma that occurs during therapeutic plasma exchange (TPE) results in the nonselective removal of all plasma constituents, whether harmful or beneficial. A typical TPE removes approximately 150 g of plasma proteins (110 g of albumin and 40 g of globulin) in order to eliminate 1 to 2 g of pathologic substance.[1] This bulk removal requires the use of a replacement fluid, usually 5% albumin, fresh frozen plasma, or cryosupernatant-poor plasma. Five percent albumin, the safest and most commonly used fluid, is not a true physiologic replacement fluid because it does not contain the entire spectrum of plasma proteins removed. The latter two fluids have the potential to trigger life-threatening reactions (eg, transfusion-related acute lung injury) and transmit viral infections.

In a TPE using 5% albumin as a replacement fluid, significant decreases in clotting factors occur. The majority of factor levels return to normal within 4 to 24 hours after completion of the procedure. An exception is fibrinogen, which reaches only 66% of the baseline level by 72 hours after completion of the procedure.[2] As a result, a risk of bleeding, which increases with serial procedures, exists in hemostatically challenged patients following TPE. Five percent albumin is devoid of immunoglobulins, and albumin exchanges lead to significant reductions in immunoglobulin levels with a theoretical risk of infection when patients undergo long courses of TPE.[2] Finally, the albumin present in 5% albumin solutions cannot fulfill some physiologic functions because the drug and metabolite-binding sites are occupied by sodium caprylate and other preservatives necessary for its storage.[1]

Because of these disadvantages inherent in TPE, methods have been developed to selectively remove pathologic plasma components with the "cleansed" plasma being returned to the patient. This minimizes the depletion of normal plasma constituents and avoids exposure to replacement fluids. The major disadvantage of such procedures is the expense involved, as the components of the selective removal systems cost significantly more than the albumin replacement fluid.

All selective removal procedures currently available in the United States require an initial step in which plasma is separated from the cellular elements of whole blood, either by filtration or centrifugation. The separated plasma is then perfused through a selective removal column or filter, and the treated plasma is recombined with the cellular components and re-infused.

Selective removal columns may be either single-use or multi-use columns. Once single-use columns become saturated, they are discarded. In this setting, the total amount of substance that can be removed is limited by the column size and sorbent capacity. Columns that can be used multiple times can be regenerated. They are perfused with an eluant buffer that removes the bound target substance, freeing the binding sites so that the column can be used to treat additional plasma. With columns that can be regenerated, the amount of plasma that can be treated is theoretically unlimited.

LDL Apheresis

Introduction and Accepted Indications

The selective removal of low-density lipoproteins (LDL) is referred to as LDL apheresis. These procedures are performed on individuals with familial hypercholesterolemia who are either heter - ozygous or homozygous for genes encoding abnormal LDL receptors that limit hepatic clearance of apolipoprotein B-100-containing molecules, such as LDL, from the circulation. This results in accelerated atherosclerosis and premature death due to cardiac disease. Individuals homozygous for a defective receptor will develop soft tissue collections of cholesterol called xanthomas by age 4 years and die from coronary artery disease by age 20 years. Heterozygotes will develop xanthomas by age 20 years and atherosclerosis by age 30 years. All homozygotes and a portion of heterozygotes fail to respond satisfactorily to dietary and medical management of the elevated LDL cholesterol.[3]

Criteria approved by the Food and Drug Administration (FDA) for the selection of patients to undergo LDL apheresis are given in Table 17.[4] Numerous series have examined the outcomes of patients treated with LDL apheresis and found that 75% to 83% of the patients demonstrate improvement or stabilization of their coronary artery atherosclerosis after long-term treatment.[5] These studies have demonstrated significant reductions in cholesterol, regression of xanthomas, disappearance of electrocardiogram (EKG) abnormalities, regression of coronary artery lesions, improvement in exercise tolerance, and prolongation of life span.[6] Familial hypercholesterolemia is a standard and accepted primary indication (Category I) for LDL apheresis according to the American Society for Apheresis (ASFA)[7] and AABB.[8]

A typical patient can be managed with a single treatment every 2 weeks because of the relatively long half-life of LDL. For new patients or those who fail to respond to this regimen, more frequent procedures may be necessary (eg, weekly). In those with good response, less frequent treatment may be possible. The total volume of plasma treated with each procedure depends on the type of LDL apheresis instrument used.

Table 17. Patient Criteria for the Use of LDL Apheresis in Hypercholesterolemia[4]

- Homozygotes with an LDL cholesterol ≥500 mg/dL
- Heterozygotes with an LDL cholesterol ≥300 mg/dL*
- Heterozygotes with an LDL cholesterol ≥200 mg/dL and documented coronary artery disease*

*For heterozygotes, a 6-month trial of maximal drug therapy in combination with an American Heart Association Step II diet is to be tried before initiating therapy.

Dextran Sulfate LDL Apheresis

Dextran sulfate absorption (Liposorber LA-15, Kaneka, Osaka, Japan) is currently approved by the FDA for use in the United States. In this method, plasma is separated from whole blood using a hollow fiber separator. The separated plasma is pumped through a column containing dextran sulfate bound to cellulose beads. In the column, the negatively charged dextran sulfate interacts with the positively charged apolipoprotein B-100 on the LDL, binding the LDL to the column. Treated plasma is then mixed with the cellular elements of the blood and returned to the patient.[5]

In this system, two dextran sulfate columns are used for each procedure. The first column becomes saturated after processing a defined amount of plasma, at which time the Liposorber LA-15 instrument automatically switches flow to a second column. The first column is regenerated by rinsing it with 4.1% NaCl. The eluted LDL and hypertonic saline solution are collected into a waste bag. Following regeneration, the column is perfused with a solution of normal saline and heparin and is then ready to treat additional plasma. A salinometer monitors the fluid leaving the column in order to prevent infusion of hypertonic saline into the patient. Heparin is routinely used as the anticoagulant for this procedure and is administered by an integral heparin pump present in the instrument.[5] The advantages and disadvantages of this system, along with the effects of treatment on cholesterol levels, are given in Table 18.

This system has an extracorporeal volume of 400 mL. As a result, caution should be used when treating children with this device. The instrument operator's manual specifically warns against treating patients with a body weight less than 15 kg and patients less than 5 years of age.[12]

Heparin-Induced Extracorporeal LDL Precipitation

Heparin-induced extracorporeal LDL precipitation (HELP) (Plasmat Secura, B. Braun Medical, Bethlehem, PA) was the second method for LDL apheresis to be approved by the FDA for use in the United States. With this instrument, plasma is also separated from whole blood using a hollow fiber separator. The separated

Table 18. Comparison of Currently Available LDL Apheresis Systems[5,9-11]

	Method of LDL Removal	Substances Removed	Advantages	Disadvantages
Dextran sulfate (Liposorber LA-15, Kaneka, Osaka, Japan)	Binding to dextran sulfate based upon electrical charge	LDL – 56% to 65% HDL – 9% to 30% Triglycerides – 34% to 40% Lp(a) – 52% to 61%	Column can be regenerated	– Requires plasma separation – High hematocrit may interfere with plasma separation
HELP (Plasmat Secura, B. Braun Medical, Bethlehem, PA)	Precipitation of LDL by heparin at an acidic pH	LDL – 67% HDL – 15% Triglycerides – 41% Lp(a) – 62%	Removes fibrinogen	– High hematocrit may interfere with plasma separation – Complicated system

(Continued)

Table 18. Comparison of Currently Available LDL Apheresis Systems[5,9-11] **(Continued)**

	Method of LDL Removal	Substances Removed	Advantages	Disadvantages
Membrane differential filtration apheresis	Separation based on size by filtering plasma with a second filter	LDL – 56% HDL – 25% Triglycerides – 49% Lp(a) – 53%	Removes fibrinogen	– High hematocrit may interfere with plasma separation – Loss of some albumin, HDL, and IgG
Immunoadsorption (Plasmaselect, Teterow, Germany)	Immobilized sheep apolipoprotein B-100 antibodies	LDL – 64% HDL – 14% Triglycerides – 42% Lp(a) – 64%	Column can be regenerated	– Exposure to animal proteins
Lipoprotein hemoperfusion (DALI, Fresenius HemoCare, Redmond, WA)	Binding to polyacrylate-coated polyacrylamide beads based on electrical charge	LDL – 61% HDL – 30% Triglycerides – 42% Lp(a) – 64%	Plasma separation is not necessary	Column cannot be regenerated

plasma is mixed with a sodium acetate buffer (pH 4.84) containing heparin. The molecules containing apolipoprotein B-100 form an insoluble precipitate in the presence of heparin at the lowered pH. This precipitate is then removed by filtration. The heparin is subsequently adsorbed from the plasma by a diethylaminoethyl cellulose filter, and the acetate and extra volume that were added to the plasma are removed through bicarbonate dialysis/ultrafiltration. The treated plasma is then combined with the cellular elements and returned to the patient.[5] The advantages and disadvantages of this system, along with the effects of treatment on cholesterol levels, are given in Table 18.

Other LDL Apheresis Systems Available Outside the United States

Three additional systems (membrane differential filtration apheresis, immunoadsorption, and lipoprotein hemoperfusion) are available outside the United States for the removal of LDL cholesterol. Their advantages, disadvantages, mechanisms of action, and effects on cholesterol levels are summarized in Table 18.

Reactions to LDL Apheresis

Bambauer et al[5] reviewed 4330 LDL apheresis procedures, including all of the techniques listed in Table 18. They found a reaction rate of 10.9%.[5] The majority of these reactions were mild, with no differences between the type and frequency of reactions among the different systems examined. The most common side effects reported were posttreatment bleeding (3.5%), vomiting (2.5%), hypoglycemia (2.4%), hypotension (2.2%), allergic reactions (0.2%), and shock (0.1%).[5]

The use of angiotensin-converting enzyme (ACE) inhibitors by patients being treated with the dextran sulfate column is an important consideration. Concurrent treatment with ACE inhibitors is associated with reactions consisting of flushing, hypotension, bradycardia, and dyspnea. These reactions result from activation of the kinin system by the negatively charged dextran sulfate in the column. This generates bradykinin, which under normal circumstances is rapidly inactivated by kininase I and II. ACE inhibitors, however, block the actions of these enzymes, allowing high levels of bradykinin to accumulate and cause the symptoms described.[13] These reactions can be avoided by ensuring that the patient is taking a short-acting ACE inhibitor (eg, lisinopril) and withholding the medication for 24 hours before dextran sulfate LDL apheresis treatment. Alternatively, the patient can be switched to another medication such as an angiotensin receptor blocker (eg, losartan). If other ACE inhibitors are used, the necessary interval after the last dose should be based on the half-life of the agent. In the study by Bambauer et al, patients taking ACE inhibitors were not treated with LDL apheresis.[5]

Other Indications for LDL Apheresis

Refsum's disease is a rare metabolic disorder characterized by the inability to metabolize dietary phytanic acid. Phytanic acid accumulates and is bound to lipoproteins as well as adipose tissue. This disorder is characterized by severe neurologic symptoms that worsen during periods of adipose tissue turnover: for example, during illness or weight loss. There have been reports of the use of membrane differential filtration apheresis to remove lipoproteins and thereby deplete the excess phytanic acid circulating in the plasma.[13] Theoretically, all forms of LDL apheresis should be effective in treating this disease.

There have also been reports of the treatment of small numbers of patients with some LDL apheresis systems in which the removal of cholesterol is not the only goal of treatment. With these systems, the treatments remove other plasma components, such as fibrinogen, in addition to cholesterol. It has been hypothesized that removal of these large macromolecules might result in an alteration of blood flow characteristics that would enhance flow to compromised end organs. LDL apheresis instruments are currently being evaluated for the treatment of acute stroke (HELP), acute myocardial ischemia (HELP), sudden sensorineural hearing loss (HELP), peripheral arterial occlusive disease (dextran sulfate), and age-related macular degeneration (membrane differential filtration apheresis).[5]

170

Staphylococcal Protein A Immunoadsorption Columns

Overview

Staphylococcal protein A is a bacterial cell wall component that can bind to the Fc portion of IgG. In addition, it can bind to certain inherited regions of the Fab portion of the heavy chain, resulting in an ability to bind non-IgG immunoglobulins to a lesser extent.[14] Staphylococcal protein A binds strongly to IgG1, IgG2, and IgG4 but only variably to IgG3, IgM, and IgA. This ability to bind to immunoglobulins has been used to create selective removal columns to treat diseases resulting from the presence of pathologic antibodies. Two types of staphylococcal protein A columns are available: the staphylococcal protein A-silica (PAS) column (Prosorba, Fresenius HemoCare, Redmond, WA) and the staphylococcal protein A-agarose (PAA) column (Immunosorba, Fresenius HemoCare). For both columns, the patient's plasma is separated from the cellular elements by a centrifugal apheresis instrument or membrane plasma separator. The plasma is then perfused through a protein A column, recombined with the cellular elements, and returned to the patient.

Staphylococcal Protein A-Silica Column (Prosorba)

The PAS column consists of staphylococcal protein A bound to silica beads. Once saturated, the column cannot be regenerated and must be discarded, limiting the amount of plasma that can be treated to 2 liters.[14] The total amount of immunoglobulin removed by treating this volume of plasma can be as little as 1 g of native IgG and 100 mg of immunoglobulin in circulating immune complexes (CICs).[1]

The mechanism of action of the PAS column is not well understood. The column removes free immunoglobulin as well as CICs; however, the total amount of immunoglobulins and complexes removed is very small—smaller than would be removed by a single TPE treatment—and would not explain a beneficial effect of the procedure. It is hypothesized that treatment with the

PAS column produces immune modulation that allows the immune system to respond better to the underlying disorder. A number of mechanisms for immune modulation have been proposed; however, none has yet been proven. The presence of small circulating immune complexes (CICs) might induce immune suppression; such complexes are less readily removed by the reticuloendothelial system, and their presence might predispose to an excess of antigen relative to antibody that might in turn induce a state of immune paralysis toward the antigen in question. By removing small CICs, the PAS column might relieve the antigen excess situation and reduce the supposed immune suppression. Alternatively, beneficial effects have been proposed to be caused by the activation of the complement cascade that accompanies binding of IgG to staphylococcal protein A. The complement fragments generated thereby, which would then be infused into the patient when the treated plasma is reinfused, might activate the immune system, resulting in correction of an immune imbalance. Also, staphylococcal protein A is a T- and B-cell mitogen. Some protein A is eluted from the column during a treatment, and the infusion of protein A into the patient upon reinfusion of treated plasma could result in T- and B-cell proliferation and immune system activation. Autoantibody production is thought by some to be regulated by anti-idiotypic antibodies that recognize antigen-binding sites on the Fab portion of autoantibodies, thereby blocking their ability to bind to target antigen and silencing the autoimmune response. Treatment with the PAS column has been shown to result in an increase in anti-idiotypic antibodies, which could then dampen the autoimmune response. This increase in anti-idiotypic antibodies could be the result of changes in autoantibody conformation and/or in immune complex size that might enhance the immunogenicity of these antibodies.[15] Finally, recent evidence suggests that staphylococcal protein A leached from the column may induce targeted B-cell deletion by activating apoptotic pathways among B cells expressing the immunoglobulin V_H3 gene family. B cells expressing this gene family have been shown to be involved in autoantibody production in immune thrombocytopenic purpura (ITP) and rheumatoid arthritis, the two diseases for which treatment with the PAS column has been found to be beneficial.[16]

Thus, multiple mechanisms have been proposed to explain putative immune modulation by the PAS column; however, the true mechanism or mechanisms behind any beneficial effect of the column remain to be elucidated.

FDA-Approved Indications for the PAS Column

There are two FDA-approved indications for the use of the PAS columns—ITP refractory to standard therapy and rheumatoid arthritis.

ITP is an autoimmune disorder characterized by thrombocytopenia with episodes of bleeding in the presence of normal or increased numbers of megakaryocytes. It is associated with IgG autoantibodies toward platelet glycoproteins. These antibodies coat platelets, resulting in their removal by the reticuloendothelial system. Standard therapies include corticosteroids, other immunomodulatory drugs, and splenectomy. The PAS column has been used to treat patients who fail to respond to this standard therapy. In studies of patients with refractory ITP who received off-line treatments of as little as 250 mL of plasma, 50% responded with increases in platelet counts following six treatments over 2 to 3 weeks. The median time to response was 2 weeks. Those responding demonstrated reductions in platelet-associated IgG and CICs.[15] Because of these studies, the PAS column is approved by the FDA for the treatment of ITP refractory to standard therapy.[14] The use of PAS columns to treat refractory ITP is considered to be a generally accepted supportive or adjunct therapy (Category II indication) by ASFA[7] and AABB.[8]

Rheumatoid arthritis is an autoimmune condition characterized by severe inflammatory joint disease and a number of systemic manifestations. CICs and rheumatoid factors have been implicated in the disease process. A randomized, double-blind, sham-controlled trial of the use of the PAS column in patients failing to respond to methotrexate or at least two other disease-modifying drugs has been published. After 12 weekly treatments, 31.9% of the treated patients improved compared with 11.4% of the control patients.[15] Because of this and other studies, the PAS column is approved by the FDA for the treatment of rheumatoid arthritis.[14] The use of PAS columns to treat rheumatoid arthritis is considered to be a generally accepted supportive or adjunct therapy (Category II indication) by ASFA[7] and AABB.[8]

Adverse Reactions to the PAS Column

Side effects seen with the PAS column include fever and chills, nausea, vomiting, pain, hypotension, dyspnea, allergic reactions, headache, hypertension, and tachycardia. Such reactions have been reported to occur in 34% of procedures.[17]

These effects may result from a number of mechanisms. As mentioned, the PAS columns activate the complement cascade, generating complement fragments such as C5a. These substances can produce anaphylactoid reactions and could explain the allergic and hypotensive reactions seen in some patients. In the manufacture of the original PAS columns, there was contamination of the columns with lipopolysaccharide (endotoxin). Infusion of this, as well as leached staphylococcal protein A, could also produce reactions such as hypotension and fever.[17]

Most reactions seen with PAS columns are mild, starting up to 1 hour after treatment and lasting 1 to 2 hours; however, severe reactions, including death, have been reported. The four patterns of severe reactions seen with the PAS column include anaphylaxis, vasculitis, large vessel thrombosis, and exacerbations of underlying disease.[17] Because of the increased incidence of thrombosis in patients treated with the PAS column, especially those with rheumatoid arthritis, the manufacturer lists as contraindications 1) a history or evidence of a hypercoagulable state as well as pre-existing abnormalities of coagulation, including anything that may precipitate a thrombotic event, or 2) a history of a thromboembolic event.[18] In patients being treated for rheumatoid arthritis, the manufacturer also recommends the daily administration of aspirin throughout the 12-week course of treatment.[18] As with the dextran sulfate LDL apheresis columns, patients taking ACE inhibitors can experience unopposed bradykinin effects.

Staphylococcal Protein A-Agarose Column (Immunosorba)

The PAA column differs from the PAS column in that it can be regenerated. Each column contains staphylococcal protein A bound to agarose beads. Plasma is perfused through a column until it is saturated with 1.25 to 1.5 g of IgG.[1] When a column is saturated, plasma flow is switched to a second column while the first column is perfused with an eluant buffer (pH 2.2) that removes the bound immunoglobulin. The eluant buffer is then washed out of the column with a pH 7.0 buffer, and the column is then available to treat additional plasma. The ability to regenerate a pair of columns theoretically allows an unlimited volume of plasma to be treated but requires the use of a separate monitoring system (Citem 10, Fresenius HemoCare) to control plasma, eluant, and neutral buffer flow during regeneration of the columns and to prevent infusion of any eluant buffer to the patient. The PAA columns can be reused for up to 20 treatment sessions for the same patient.[14] The PAA columns cannot be used to treat different patients because of the danger of blood-borne pathogen transmission from one patient to another. Between treatment sessions, a thimerosal-containing preservative is placed into the columns and they are refrigerated.

The treatment of 2.5 plasma volumes with the PAA column results in a reduction of 97% of IgG1, 98% of IgG2, 40% of IgG3, 77% of IgG4, 56% of IgM, and 55% of IgA. Levels of albumin, fibrinogen, and antithrombin are reduced by 40%.[1]

The mechanism of action of the PAA column is thought to be due solely to the removal of immunoglobulins.[14] As with the PAS column, however, recent evidence suggests that B-cell depletion through apoptosis may be involved.[16]

FDA-Approved Indications for the PAA Column

The PAA column is currently approved by the FDA, under a humanitarian device exemption, solely for the treatment of Factor VIII and Factor IX inhibitors. Congenital hemophilia results from an inherited deficiency of either Factor VIII (hemophilia A) or

Factor IX (hemophilia B). The absence of the factor results in a bleeding diathesis that can be effectively treated by infusions of an appropriate factor concentrate. Approximately 15% to 35% of patients with hemophilia A will develop IgG4 antibodies directed against Factor VIII, while 1% to 3% of those with hemophilia B will develop IgG4 antibodies to Factor IX. In the presence of low-titer inhibitors, higher doses of factor concentrates can be given during a bleeding episode to overcome these alloantibodies. When this fails, products containing activated coagulation factor concentrates (eg, prothrombin complex concentrates or Factor VIIa) can be given to bypass the inhibitor and achieve hemostasis. Long-term, these inhibitors can be suppressed by chronic administration of the appropriate factor concentrate to induce immune tolerance.

In addition to the alloimmune inhibitors described above, autoantibodies can develop in patients with normal genes and previously normal factor levels. The latter induce an "acquired hemophilia." Again, high-dose factor concentrates and/or activated coagulation factor concentrates can be given to treat bleeding episodes. Individuals with inhibitors are also treated with corticosteroids and cytotoxic agents in an attempt to stop production of the autoantibody. When used alone, these immunosuppressive treatments are not effective for alloantibodies produced in congenital Hemophilia A and B.

The PAA column has been used successfully to treat congenital hemophiliacs with high-titer inhibitors who fail to respond to standard therapy, as well as individuals with acquired hemophilia caused by autoantibodies to Factor VIII or Factor IX.[14] Because of the high cost associated with the doses of factor concentrates necessary to overcome inhibitors, either to stop bleeding or to aid in tolerance induction, the use of the PAA columns in this setting is one of the few instances in which selective removal columns are less expensive than the alternative therapy.[14] To induce tolerance, the PAA column is used in conjunction with cytotoxic chemotherapy, high-dose factor infusion, and/or intravenous immune globulin (IVIG). Neither ASFA nor AABB has categorized the use of the PAA column for the treatment of coagulation factor inhibitors.

Side effects associated with the PAA column include musculo-skeletal pain, nausea, vomiting, and hypotension. Approximately 26% to 30% of procedures are affected by these reactions.[17] The same mechanisms postulated to explain the reactions to the PAS column apply to the PAA column, although contamination with lipopolysaccharide (endotoxin) has not been reported. As with the PAS column, most reactions are mild; however, severe reactions, including death, have been reported. Severe reactions are less common with the PAA columns than with the PAS columns.[17] As with the PAS column, patients on ACE inhibitors can experience unopposed bradykinin effects.

A unique problem that has been reported with the PAA column is the occurrence of mercury poisoning. Cases of mercury poisoning have occurred when the thimerosal-containing preservative was not removed from the columns before use and was therefore infused into the patient. In addition, recent cases of elevated mercury levels have been reported in patients undergoing large numbers of treatments with properly pre-rinsed columns.

Other Indications for Staphylococcal Protein A Columns

Additional diseases that have been treated off-label with the PAA and PAS columns are listed in Table 19. Only limited numbers of patients have been treated with the PAA and/or PAS columns in these settings. The use of staphylococcal protein A columns for these disorders has not been classified by ASFA or AABB.

Membrane Differential Filtration

Description and Indications

Membrane differential filtration apheresis, also called cascade filtration apheresis or double filtration apheresis, is a method for the selective removal of plasma components based on size of the mol-

Table 19. Other Disorders Treated with Staphylococcal Protein A Columns*[14,15]

PAS Column (Prosorba)	PAA Column (Immunosorba)
Antiglomerular basement membrane disease (Goodpasture's syndrome)	Chemotherapy-induced thrombotic thrombocytopenic purpura (eg, mitomycin-C)
Wegner's granulomatosis	Platelet alloimmunization
Focal segmental glomerulosclerosis	Solid organ malignancy
Systemic lupus erythematosus	Paraneoplastic syndromes
Myasthenia gravis	Paraprotein-associated polyneuropathy
Acute demyelinating polyneuropathy (Guillain-Barré syndrome)	Autoimmune hemolytic anemia
Humoral rejection of solid organs	

*Off-label uses not approved by the FDA.

ecules.[19] Whole blood is separated into the cellular elements and plasma by an initial filtration step using a plasma separator. The plasma is then filtered through a second filter with a smaller pore size that allows the passage of albumin and smaller molecules but retains larger molecules such as immunoglobulins, lipoproteins, and immune complexes.[19] While not as selective as some of the procedures described earlier, membrane differential filtration apheresis can still be performed without replacement fluids because albumin is spared. Anticoagulation for these procedures can be either heparin or citrate.

Currently, membrane differential filtration apheresis systems are not available for use in the United States outside of clinical trials. They are, however, widely used elsewhere. Membrane filtration apheresis can be used as a substitute for TPE in autoimmune disorders such as myasthenia gravis and acute inflammatory demyelinating polyneuropathy (AIDP or Guillain-Barré syndrome) that are treated in order to remove pathologic antibodies.[19] The benefit in this setting is that replacement fluids are avoided, although the clinical benefit may not be equivalent to that of TPE.[20] Because it is only semi-selective, membrane differential filtration apheresis also removes large macromolecules other than antibodies, such as fibrinogen, α_2-macroglobulin, and IgM. It has been hypothesized by some that depletion of these plasma constituents might reduce plasma viscosity, blood viscosity, erythrocyte aggregation, and platelet aggregation. This, in turn, might improve blood flow through the microcirculation. Membrane differential filtration apheresis performed with this hypothetical rationale in mind is sometimes referred to as "rheopheresis."[21]

Adverse Reactions to Membrane Differential Filtration

Yeh et al[19] reported the frequency and types of reactions among patients undergoing membrane differential filtration apheresis as an alternative to plasma exchange. Their patient population consisted predominantly of patients with autoimmune neurologic disorders. Among 2502 procedures in 335 patients, 26.3% of procedures were complicated by reactions. It should be noted that this included problems with the catheters used for vascular access, such as catheter occlusion and line infection. The most common reactions directly attributable to the procedure itself were hemolysis (20%) and hypotension (3.3%). The hemolysis noted resulted from damage to red cells during the initial plasma separation. The hemolysis seen, while identifiable to the instrument operator, was clinically insignificant, with the average decrease in hemoglobin being 0.2 g/dL.

Klingel et al[21] reported on the frequency of reactions in patients undergoing rheopheresis and found an overall frequency of reactions of 4.65% among 2021 procedures in 322 patients. The most common reactions were hypotension (2.08%), hematoma/bleeding (0.79%), and dizziness (0.59%). The majority of reactions were mild, with only 1.19% requiring intervention.

Other Selective Removal Systems

Other selective removal systems are available or in development in other countries.[22-24] Two conceptually similar systems are the Coraffin column (Fresenius HemoCare) and the Medisorba MG-50 column (Kuraray Medical Inc., Kurashiki, Japan). These contain synthetic peptides that mimic an antigenic determinant on the target antigens for autoantibodies implicated in dilated cardiomyopathy and myasthenia gravis, respectively.[23,25] These columns are truly selective in that only antibodies targeting specific antigens thought to be involved in the disease process are removed. All other immunoglobulins are returned to the patient.

Summary

Selective removal systems offer advantages over TPE, but barriers currently limit their widespread adoption. First, there have been limited numbers of clinical trials to demonstrate efficacy, especially compared with TPE. This, in turn, has resulted in limited regulatory approval for these devices in the United States, which further limits research. Finally, the costs of these systems, especially in this time of limited health-care resources, limit widespread adoption of even those systems that have received FDA approval. Despite this, the growing number of these systems holds the promise of simpler, selective treatments for a variety of diseases.

References

1. Vamvakas EC, Pineda AA. Selective extraction of plasma constituents. In: McLeod BC, Price TH, Weinstein R, eds. Apheresis: Principles and practice. 2nd ed. Bethesda, MD: AABB Press, 2003:437-76.

2. Winters JL, Pineda AA. Hemapheresis. In: Henry J, ed. Clinical diagnosis and management by laboratory methods. New York, NY: WB Saunders, 2001:776-805.

3. Goldstein JL, Hobbs HH, Brown MS. Familial hypercholesterolemia. In: Beuadet AL, Sly WS, Valle D, eds. The metabolic and molecular basis of inherited disease. New York, NY: McGraw-Hill, 1995:1981-2030.

4. Gordon B, Stein E, Jones P, Illingworth D. Indications for low-density lipoprotein apheresis. Am J Cardiol 1994; 74:1109-12.

5. Bambauer R, Schiel R, Latza R. Low-density lipoprotein apheresis: An overview. Ther Apher Dial 2003;7:382-90.

6. Bosch T, Wendler T. State of the art of low-density lipoprotein apheresis in the year 2003. Ther Apher Dial 2004; 8:76-9.

7. McLeod BC. Introduction to the third special issue: Clinical applications of therapeutic apheresis. J Clin Apheresis 2000;15:1-5.

8. Smith JW, Weinstein R, Hillyer KL, for the AABB Hemapheresis Committee. Therapeutic apheresis: A summary of current indication categories endorsed by the AABB and the American Society for Apheresis. Transfusion 2003; 43:820-2.

9. Parhofer KG, Geiss HC, Schwandt P. Efficacy of different low-density lipoprotein apheresis methods. Ther Apher 2000;4:382-5.

10. Hershcovici T, Schechner V, Orlin J, et al. Effect of different LDL-apheresis methods on parameters involved in atherosclerosis. J Clin Apheresis 2004;19:90-7.

11. Matsuda Y, Malchesky PS, Nose Y. Assessment of currently available low-density lipoprotein apheresis systems. Artif Organs 1994;18:93-9.

12. Liposorber LA-15 system operator's manual. Osaka, Japan: Kaneka, 2001.
13. Winters JL, Pineda AA, McLeod BC, Grima KM. Therapeutic apheresis in renal and metabolic diseases. J Clin Apheresis 2000;15:53-73.
14. Matic G, Bosch T, Ramlow W. Background and indications for protein A-based extracorporeal immunoadsorption. Ther Apher 2001;5:394-403.
15. Levy J, Degani N. Correcting immune imbalance: The use of Prosorba column treatment for immune disorders. Ther Apher Dial 2003;7:197-205.
16. Silverman GJ, Goodyear CS, Siegel DL. On the mechanism of staphylococcal protein A immunomodulation. Transfusion 2005;45:274-80.
17. Huestis DW, Morrison F. Adverse effects of immune adsorption with staphylococcal protein A columns. Transfus Med Rev 1996;10:62-70.
18. Prosorba protein A immunoadsorption column essential prescribing information. Redmond, WA: Fresenius HemoCare, 2001.
19. Yeh JH, Chen WH, Chiu HC. Complications of double-filtration plasmapheresis. Transfusion 2004;44:1621-5.
20. Lyu RK, Chen WH, Hsieh ST. Plasma exchange versus double filtration plasmapheresis in the treatment of Guillain-Barré syndrome. Ther Apher 2002;6:163-6.
21. Klingel R, Fassbender C, Fassbender T, et al. Rheopheresis: Rheologic, functional, and structural aspects. Ther Apher 2000;4:348-57.
22. Jansen M, Schmaldienst S, Banyai S, et al. Treatment of coagulation inhibitors with extracorporeal immunoadsorption (Ig-Therasorb). Br J Haematol 2001;112:91-7.
23. Ronspeck W, Brinckmann R, Egner R, et al. Peptide based adsorbers for therapeutic immunoadsorption. Ther Apher Dial 2003;7:91-7.
24. Ullrich H, Jakob W, Frohlich D, et al. A new endotoxin adsorber: First clinical application. Ther Apher 2001;5:326-34.
25. Nakaji S, Hayashi N. Adsorption column for myasthenia gravis treatment: Medisorba MG-50. Ther Apher Dial 2003;7:78-84.

INDEX

187

in sickle cell disease, 120-124
stiff-person syndrome, *77,*
84-85

O

Orders, physician, 16
Overdose, drug, *87,* 98, *99,* 100

P

PAA (staphylococcal protein
A-agarose) columns, 175-177
    adverse reactions, 177
    indications, 175-176
    mechanism, 175
PANDAS (pediatric autoimmune neu-
    rologic disorders associated with
    Streptococcal infections), *77,*
    150-151
Paraneoplastic cerebellar degenera-
    tion, 85
Paraneoplastic encephalomyelitis, 85
Paraneoplastic syndromes, *77,* 85,
    178
Paraprotein removal, 18
Paraprotein-associated
    polyneuropathy, *178*
Parathormone, 12
Paresthesias, 24-25, 48
Patient assessments, 13, 15
Pauci-immune rapidly progressive
    glomerulonephritis, 88
Pediatric autoimmune neurologic dis-
    orders associated with streptococ-
    cal infections (PANDAS), *77,*
    150-151
Pediatric therapeutic apheresis,
    135-158
        for acute chest syndrome, 124
        for acute hepatic failure, 97
        adverse reactions, 144-145
        anticoagulation, 137-138, 156
        for atypical TTP/HUS,
            151-152
        for familial hypercholesterol-
            emia, 153
        intravascular volume shifts,
            138-140, *141,* 142-144

leukapheresis, 135, 155-156,
    157, 158
overview, 135-136
for PANDAS, 150-151
for phytanic storage disease,
    154
plasmapheresis, 150-154
for Rasmussen's encephalitis,
    152-153
red cell balance, 139-140,
    141, 142-144
red cell exchange, 116-117,
    146-150
for red cell removal, 149-150
for sickle cell disease,
    123-124, 146-149
vascular access, 136-137
Pemphigus vulgaris, 45
Peripheral arterial occlusive disease,
    170
Peripheral intravenous catheters, 17
Peripheral neuropathy with
    monoclonal gammopathy, *77,*
    80-81
Peripherally inserted central venous
    catheters (PICC lines), 18, 137
Phenotype matching, 117, 125,
    148-149
Phlebotomy, for red cell removal,
    149-150
Photopheresis, 41-46
        for autoimmune diseases, 45
        for cutaneous T-cell lym-
            phoma, 42-43
        for graft-vs-host disease,
            43-44
        mechanism of action, 45-46
        for transplantation rejection,
            36, 44
Physician orders, 16
Phytanic acid storage disease
    apheresis for, 170
    in children, 154
    therapeutic plasma exchange
        for, *77,* 100-101
PICC lines, 18, 137
Plasma, Cryoprecipitate Reduced, 62,
    63